THE LOVELACE MEDICAL CENTER

THE LOVELACE MEDICAL CENTER

Pioneer in American Health Care

by Jake W. Spidle, Jr.

UNIVERSITY OF NEW MEXICO PRESS
Albuquerque

Library of Congress Cataloging-in-Publication Data

Spidle, Jake W., 1941–
The Lovelace Medical Center.

Bibliography: p.
Includes index.
1. Lovelace Medical Center—History. 3. Lovelace Medical Foundation—History. I. Title. [DNLM: 1. Lovelace Medical Center. 2. Academies and Institutes —history—New Mexico. WA 24 L898S]
RA982.A313L687 1987 362.1'1'0978961 87-10250
ISBN 0-8263-1007-9

Design by Susan Gutnik

First edition.

For Christopher, Susan, and Joseph, with much love

Contents

Preface

In the spring of 1967, eighty-three-year-old Dr. William Randolph Lovelace I was physically ailing and still suffering from the shock of the tragic death eighteen months earlier of his nephew and successor Dr. William Randolph Lovelace II. But the convictions that had oriented his life remained unchanged. In a letter of advice and encouragement to a teenaged grand-nephew away at military school, he wrote,

> What you must do, Kelly, is try your hardest and prepare yourself as best you can, then look around for a place to serve. That's what I was trying to do when I started this place [the Lovelace Clinic] so many years ago.

In the sixty-five years that have passed since the founding of the Lovelace Clinic in 1922, the institution created by the country doctor became "a place to serve" for several thousand health care professionals and one of the premier medical institutions of the West. In the process it established a tradition of pioneering as well, a tradition which has become perhaps the most distinctive aspect of the Albuquerque medical center's history. The list of pioneering achievements or ventures associated with the place is a long one. It was an innovator in the establishment of medical group practice in the Southwest; a trailblazer in bringing specialty medicine to the region; the earliest and largest-scaled medical foundation involved in medical education and research in the entire Southwest; a national and international pioneer in the modern field of aviation and space medicine; a world renowned leader in inhalation toxicology research and other bioenvironmental research spheres; a pathfinder in development of modern health-delivery systems, such as health maintenance organizations (HMOs) and satellite clinic operations; a forerunner in the training of modern physician-executives for successful competition in the world of 21st century corporate medicine; a challenger of tradition in the incorporation of modern marketing tools and strategies within the world of medicine; and much else could be cited within the surprisingly creative and flexible record of the Albuquerque institution. Dr. Lovelace's "place to serve" became that and much more. It indelibly set its stamp on the development of health care in the Southwest and, beyond that, several of its innovations have attracted national and international attention. As a matter of fact, since 1970 the Lovelace name may even be said to have an extraterrestrial extension. In December of that year, the National Aeronautics and Space Administration announced that a crater on the moon had been named in honor of Dr. William Randolph Lovelace II, a space medicine pioneer and cofounder of the Lovelace Foundation.

This book is intended to do two things. It is meant, obviously, to honor this important Southwestern institution in the year of several anniversaries important to it—the sixty-fifth of the Lovelace Clinic, the fortieth of the Lovelace Medical Foundation, and the thirty-fifth of the Lovelace Medical Center hospital—and the men and women who envisioned its service, charted its course, and labored to fulfill its goals. It is also intended to fix the history of the Lovelace institution within the general history of the community and region it has served and to integrate its development within the broader history of American medicine in the twentieth century. It has earned consideration of that sort through many decades now of contribution to its region and to medicine in general.

Albuquerque, N.M.
February 1987

Acknowledgments

IN RESEARCHING AND WRITING this book, I have received the full cooperation and support of the Lovelace institution. The people now on its staff and many of those who served it in the past have opened all doors to me, made available everything I wanted to examine, and ransacked their memories when I couldn't get pieces of the story to fit together just right from the documents. They were eager to have the Lovelace story told, for they are proud of the institution and convinced its story deserved the telling. At the same time, I was encouraged "to let the chips fall where they may," and I have tried very hard to look at the Lovelace center from "outside the house."

All the agencies and individuals who helped move the Lovelace history project forward cannot be mentioned by name here. Particular thanks are due to the Board of Trustees of the Lovelace Medical Foundation who valued this effort enough to make it a special project of the board and who generously supported its work. At the individual level, special thanks are due first of all to Dr. Mel Twiest, general surgeon and vice-chairman of the clinic's Board of Governors, and Dr. Waneta Tuttle, physiologist and vice president-chief operating officer of the foundation. Though relative youngsters themselves within the Lovelace operation, they sensed the need for the institution to take a close look at its roots to help orient the place in a time of rapid change. Without exception they have consistently and willingly gone to bat for the history project, and their support has been central to its success. Similarly, from within the Lovelace administration Merle Tucker has capably steered the work from its very start—giving good advice, handling all the logistical arrangements necessary to keep the project on track, and never wavering in his conviction of the work's importance. To the degree this history has solidity and merit, I hope these three people will share the credit. Special mention ought also be made of the help rendered by Drs. Sam White, Don Kilgore, David Ottensmeyer, and Derick Pasternak, each of whom made available large chunks of time to help me in understanding the Lovelace institution by providing their perspectives on it. In addition, there are some forty other Lovelace physicians, administrators, trustees, and others who gave their time and insights in my effort to put together a comprehensive story. To all of them I here extend my sincere thanks and appreciation.

Joe Foster and his co-workers in the Lovelace Photography Department, especially Phil Hadley and Karla McKitrick, are responsible for most of the illustrations used in this book and several times went far out of their way in helping me to photodocument this study. Jeane Strub and Mary Strawn of the Lovelace Library assisted in directing me to materials and in answering many questions, while Tommie Britton in her customary deft and efficient way resolved miscellaneous and sundry problems encountered along the way. Mildred Morgan of the Inhalation Toxicology Research Institute; Janet Johnson, Judith DuCharme, Kathy Mondragon, and Lillian Croghan of the Medical Center Library at the University of New Mexico; Linda Lewis at the General Library of the University of New Mexico; Michelle McGinnis, formerly of the State Board of Medical Examiners' office; and Bob Dauner of the Museum of Albuquerque all deserve my thanks and appreciation. Special thanks, once again, to Dr. Peter Olch of the Uniformed Services University of the Health Sciences, Bethesda, Maryland, for his good counsel and encouragement. And, as always, to my wife and children, my deep appreciation for their patience and support.

ONE

Lovelace and Lassetter

WHEN THE YOUNG DOCTOR FROM MISSOURI first saw them, the plains of eastern New Mexico Territory were just beginning to bloom. Only a few years earlier, the high, dry grasslands had been the exclusive preserve of nomadic Comanches and trail-driving cowboys. A handful of Hispanic farm families clustered in the few river valleys. The southern part of the region began to develop first, with the Pecos Valley Railroad pushing northward along the Pecos River in the 1890s. The railroad linked the New Mexico towns of Eddy (later Carlsbad) and Roswell to the outside world, and a turn-of-the-century line tied the southern region to Amarillo in the cattle country of Texas. The central part of the river valley—from around Santa Rosa to Roswell—did not begin to develop rapidly until the first years of the new century, when the Atchison, Topeka and Santa Fe Railroad started construction of the Belen Cutoff.

The Santa Fe railroad had first pushed across New Mexico in the 1880s, but the main line from Raton to Belen, passing through Las Vegas and Albuquerque, was bedeviled with a host of problems. Among other things, traffic on that line had to negotiate high mountain passes at Raton and Glorieta. (Raton Pass at 7834 feet and Glorieta Pass at 7509 feet remain today the highest points in the Santa Fe system.) In the 1890s, railroad officials began to consider a more southerly route, branching off from the main line at Newton, Kansas, proceeding through Oklahoma, Texas, and eastern New Mexico, and rejoining the main line at Belen. The new route was intended to ensure a faster trip through the Southwest and to reduce wear and tear on expensive engines and other valuable equipment by avoiding the northern mountain terrain. Construction crews began to push the tracks east from Belen in 1902, and the region pierced by the cutoff began to prosper. As existing towns grew, new ones sprang up, with Clovis, founded in 1906, becoming the most prominent. Settlers moved into the countryside near the tracks, and eastern New Mexico suddenly emerged as one of the territory's most dynamic regions.

One of the new residents was a young physician, Dr. William Randolph Lovelace, who settled in the railroad camp of Sunnyside, New Mexico, in April 1906. Although he was a country boy, born in a log cabin in Belle, Missouri (population: 110), in 1883, he had not originally intended to join the population surge to the plains of frontier New Mexico. After finishing medical school, he had probably planned to return to the rural Missouri of his youth. Instead, he found himself starting his medical career in the utterly unfamiliar surroundings of frontier New Mexico, in a circumstance seemingly determined for him. Neither wanderlust nor the excitement and challenge of a newly developing land drew twenty-two-year-old Dr. Lovelace to New Mexico; rather, it was the disease that doctors of the nineteenth century called the white plague, or consumption. A case of pulmonary tuberculosis, his own, brought the Missourian west in 1906 to chase the cure in the high, dry, and sunny climate of New Mexico. It was an inauspicious, threatening start to a distinguished medical career that eventually extended over a full sixty-two years in his adopted land.

There was little, if anything, that was exceptional in the background of the tubercular young emigrant to the Southwest. His family was of modest, farmer stock, although his father had enough education to qualify as a part-time country school teacher. The young doctor's basic education was described, in later life, as "obtained largely in private schools,"[1] almost surely a polite euphemism for the spotty, catch-as-catch-can oppor-

1. Ellis Arthur Davis, ed., *The Historical Encyclopedia of New Mexico* (Albuquerque: New Mexico Historical Association, 1945), 1:324.

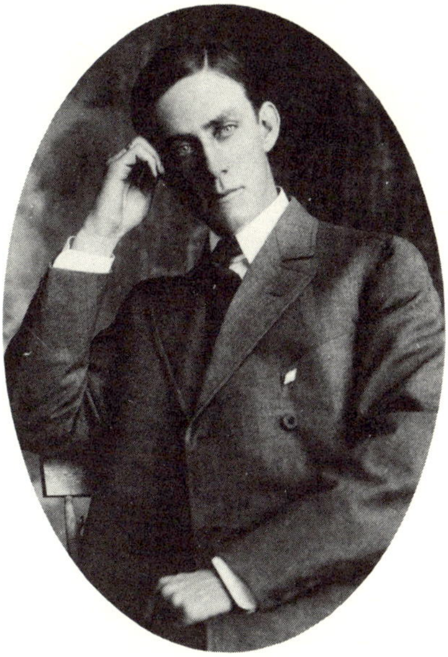

William Randolph Lovelace I as a medical student in 1903. He was a charter member of Lamda Chapter, Phi Beta Pi fraternity, the first medical fraternity at St. Louis University.

tunities available to a rural Missouri farmboy in the 1890s. Whatever enlightenment and inspiration he may or may not have received in formal school settings, he was definitely inspired by the example and encouragement of the country doctor who cared for his family during his boyhood. As a result, he left the farm country of his youth in 1902, moving to St. Louis, a hundred miles to the east, to study medicine. So far as is known, the nineteen-year-old farmboy had no formal preparation for medical school beyond a limited country school education, a circumstance not unusual for the times.

During the first years of the twentieth century, St. Louis possessed no fewer than seven different medical schools, including two or three of the most disgraceful diploma mills ever to lay claim to the title *medical school*.[2] Demonstrating the perspicacity and good judgment which were to mark his career, young Lovelace sorted through the options available and de-

2. On St. Louis medical institutions at the turn of the century, see Samuel D. Soule, *Medicine in St. Louis Medical Schools in the 19th Century* (n.p. [St. Louis]: William Washington Graves Lecture Series, 1978).

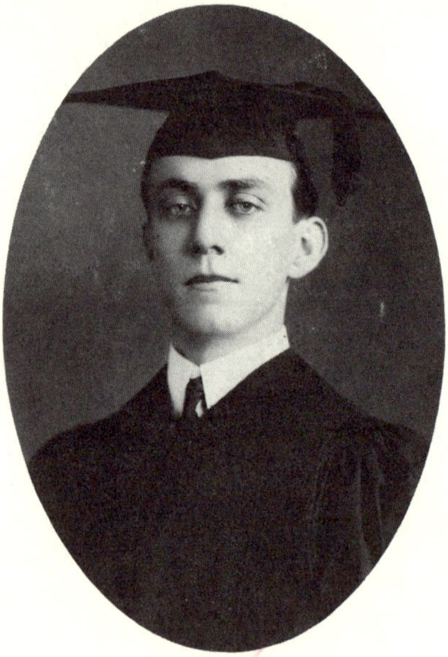

Dr. Lovelace's graduation portrait, upon completion of St. Louis University's School of Medicine in 1905.

cided upon Marion-Sims-Beaumont Medical College, one of the better schools of the city. The year after he started his three-year medical curriculum, Marion-Sims-Beaumont was absorbed within the still stronger St. Louis University School of Medicine, and it was from the latter institution that Lovelace received his medical degree in 1905.[3] After graduation, he began a one-year internship at St. Mary's Hospital in St. Louis, a large general hospital run by the Sisters of Charity.

In the winter of that internship year, 1905–1906, he was within sight of his goal—completion of his basic medical training, preliminary to setting up his own private practice—when

3. In later years some of Dr. Lovelace's rivals, eager to disparage him, spread the rumor that he had never really graduated from medical school at all. In interviewing older doctors and other health professionals in New Mexico in the 1980s, including many who knew Dr. Lovelace personally, I heard this canard several times. When I wrote to St. Louis University, both the school's registrar and archivist in its Medical Center Library confirmed Dr. Lovelace's May 1905 graduation. (Later I found a picture of him in his graduating class.) Mary Anne Sutter, Reference Librarian, St. Louis University Medical Center Library, to the author, 30 January 1985. The point is of more than passing interest, for Dr. Lovelace's rivals may have used the "questions" regarding his education in excluding him from membership in the American College of Surgeons, a distinction he never achieved.

he suddenly found himself uncharacteristically tired and weak. At first, he tried to ignore it and pushed ahead with his regular schedule, but sometime in the early months of 1906 an episode of pulmonary hemorrhage was diagnosed as the dreaded tuberculosis and brought his internship to an end. Pulmonary tuberculosis was the number one killer of young adults in turn-of-the-century America, and medical science was essentially helpless in doing anything about it. In the latter half of the nineteenth century, however, tuberculosis specialists in Europe and America had reached the conclusion that a rest regimen at high altitudes benefited many victims, even far advanced ones in some cases.[4] As a result, increasing numbers of pale-faced, coughing pilgrims made their way to the Alps, the Adirondacks, or the Rockies. High, dry, and sunny New Mexico reaped a bountiful harvest from this development, and in the half-century from 1880 to 1930, few other factors were more important in populating the territory-state. With medical authorities touting New Mexico as "nature's sanatorium for consumptives,"[5] health seekers flocked there by the thousands, and the region rapidly developed a tuberculosis industry that was virtually second to none in the nation.[6] Young Dr. Lovelace, forced to deal with the ailment within his chest, decided to seek salvation in the mountain West.

His selection of New Mexico as a place of refuge and, hopefully, healing was no accident. Before leaving St. Louis, he made arrangements with authorities of the Santa Fe railroad and the Lantry Sharp Construction Company (which was pushing the railroad's tracks across eastern New Mexico toward Kansas) to serve as railroad and company surgeon at their Sunnyside, New Mexico, railroad camp. He had no money to sustain himself during his period of recuperation, so he prudently made what

4. On tuberculosis at the turn of the century, see Esmond R. Long, "Tuberculosis in Modern Society," *Bulletin of the History of Medicine* 27, no. 4 (1953):301–19, and Frank B. Rodgers, "The Rise and Decline of the Altitude Therapy of Tuberculosis," ibid., 43, no. 1 (1969):1–16.

5. Paul M. Carrington, "The Climate of New Mexico, Nature's Sanatorium for Consumptives," *New York Medical Journal* 86 (1907):1–10.

6. For details on this important development, see Jake W. Spidle, Jr., *Doctors of Medicine in New Mexico. A History of Health and Medical Practice, 1886–1986* (Albuquerque: University of New Mexico Press, 1986), chap. 2 and 3.

arrangements he could. Caution and a good, hardheaded business sense characterized his personal and professional career from his start in 1906 to the finish. In April 1906, the weak and dispirited young doctor left his home for an uncertain future in New Mexico Territory.

Sunnyside, New Mexico, Dr. Lovelace's place of destination, was a hastily thrown up construction camp of perhaps five-hundred people in 1906. It was located approximately eight miles north of old Fort Sumner, and had grown rapidly during the year or two prior to Dr. Lovelace's arrival. (The handful of businesses and most of the people settled around old Fort Sumner quickly deserted that location for the new railroad town, and in 1910 Sunnyside was renamed Fort Sumner.)[7] Even though the railroad promised to bring "civilization" to the region, the Pecos Valley in 1906 was still very much the old, wild West. Only a bit more than twenty years earlier, Fort Sumner's most famous resident had been one William Bonney, better known as Billy the Kid,[8] and the area's rough-and-ready traditions endured in 1906 as railroad-crew roustabouts and gun-toting cowboys mingled uneasily on the town's streets. The isolation and primitivism of the region are underscored in the terse entry for Fort Sumner in a contemporary business directory:

> Fort Sumner, Guadalupe County. Population 150, is 45 miles southeast of Puerto de Luna on the Pecos River, mail twice a week from Las Vegas, weekly from Roswell, school 4 months, banking at Las Vegas and Roswell, Catholic church services semi-annually, principal resources livestock, elevation 4,060 feet.[9]

Sunnyside-Fort Sumner was a world removed from St. Louis or even Belle, Missouri. Four decades after his arrival in that strange land, Dr. Lovelace remembered his preparations for the trip and his first experiences in the Pecos Valley:

7. Don McAlavy, "Fort Sumner Country," in *Curry County, New Mexico* (Dallas: High Plains Historical Foundation, 1978), pp. 97–99.

8. In 1881, Sheriff Pat Garrett shot and killed the Kid at old Fort Sumner, and the outlaw is buried there.

9. McAlavy, "Fort Sumner Country," p. 99.

> My first location was in the little town of Sunnyside in 1906, complete with no bank balance and only $8.00 in cash after equipping the office and getting things started. Before leaving St. Louis I decided to buy a revolver, an Iver Johnson, which cost $2.50, but it was a comforting possession. At that time, in spite of the fact that I had pulmonary tuberculosis, I started in with the Lantry Sharp Construction Company and the Santa Fe Railroad as surgeon. On the way to Sunnyside I was delayed. They were to meet me at Santa Rosa with a buckboard, but they became tired of waiting and left a team for me to drive to Sunnyside, a distance of fifty miles. I arrived in Santa Rosa at 11 p.m. and left the following morning at daybreak after an employee in the livery stable brought the team down to the Mott House and put the old tin trunk in the back end. Just before departing, I went in the back of a saloon, ate breakfast and bought some sandwiches. A drive of fifty miles in the West seemed like a great distance, so I started out, frightened and sick, with the gun in my pocket, and kept hitting the broncs on the tail. Arrival had to be before dark, otherwise the Indians and natives would capture me. During the first three hours of the trip nobody was seen. Finally, far across the prairie an object appeared that looked like a wagon. As we came close it turned out to be a freighter drawn by six mules. I thought at least I could find out if I were going in the right direction. They had said in Santa Rosa, "You can't miss the town—you stay on the main road and it will take you to Sunnyside." I came up on this party and asked if I were headed for Sunnyside. "No sabe." I said, "How far?" "No sabe." He was a Mexican and my knowledge of Spanish then was nil. So I stopped and fed my team and after eating a sandwich continued driving. Late in the afternoon, about sunset, the Pecos River came into view and the little railroad town of Sunnyside. I pulled in and they took charge of my team and after eating I was so exhausted that I went to bed.[10]

For seven good years, the transplanted Missourian lived and worked in frontier Fort Sumner. It was a time that he remem-

10. Lovelace Medical Foundation, Board of Trustees, Minutes, 25 September 1947. This was the first meeting of the board of the new Lovelace foundation, and for its members, Dr. Lovelace charmingly recounted his first few days in New Mexico.

bered afterward with much pride and affection. For one thing, his health improved markedly. He suffered a serious setback not long after his arrival in the new country, for he threw himself too fully into the vigorous, punishing schedule of the frontier doctor. Unsurprisingly, the result was a renewed siege of pulmonary hemorrhaging. However, his mother came out from Missouri to nurse him back to health, and his naturally strong constitution gradually overcame the lung weakness which had brought him west. The presence of his family undoubtedly brought him cheer, for his sense of family and allegiance to his family members was always one of the most powerful forces in his life. Within two years of Dr. Lovelace's move to New Mexico, his entire Missouri family had joined him in Fort Sumner. His mother, Edna, came to stay at the time of his breakdown in 1906, and his father, John L. Lovelace, and two younger sisters, Maybelle and Lora, joined the family the next year.[11] The family migration was completed in 1908, when older brother Edgar, two years Dr. Lovelace's senior, moved to New Mexico with his new wife Jewell. Edgar and Jewell brought with them their six-month-old son, William Randolph Lovelace II, named for his doctor-uncle, and the family unit was complete.

Throughout his tenure in Fort Sumner, Dr. Lovelace was, in essence, the town's only physician, although other doctors came and went. In addition to the town, he served a large part of the surrounding Pecos Valley countryside as well. There were nearly two dozen doctors in Portales and Clovis at the eastern edge of the valley and another ten or so in Tucumcari and Santa Rosa in the north, but few of them traveled on call into the countryside. Transitorily, communities like Melrose, Taiban, Cuervo, and others boasted a doctor or two as town fortunes rose and fell in the quick, volatile development of the eastern plains, but the unqualified success of young Dr. Lovelace in claiming for himself a big share of the practice in the mid-Pecos Valley region was unique. Bouncing across the arid landscape

11. Father Lovelace's farming and teaching interests in Missouri apparently were not of sufficient importance to keep him there. He went to work in Sunnyside (and later Albuquerque) in clerical positions for the railroad; and both father and mother lived with their physician son until their deaths in 1943 and 1940, respectively.

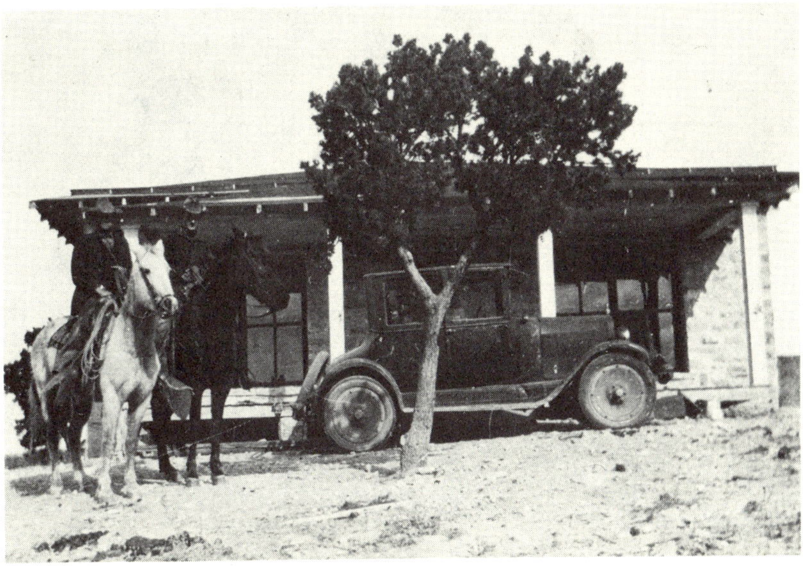

The Lovelace family homestead at Fort Sumner.

day and night in his buckboard or on horseback, he became an integral and respected part of high plains society. Attentiveness to his patients and a genuine solicitude for their well-being—qualities which over the years became legendary—were always his strong suits as a physician, and he began to build that reputation in the rough country around Fort Sumner.

His practice was the broad and varied one of the country doctor. It was focused, when circumstances allowed it, in his modest office in Fort Sumner, but even more in the homes of his patients scattered around the countryside. His first office was a crude tarpaper shack (see page 10), located adjacent to the railroad yard in Sunnyside. By 1908, the growth of his practice justified construction of a new building to house more properly the busy young professional, but a tornado quickly leveled that structure. Afterward he soon established his office in a red sandstone building which still stands and has been included on the New Mexico State Register of Cultural Properties. This building was large enough to contain several work rooms plus a drugstore, which Dr. Lovelace operated in part-

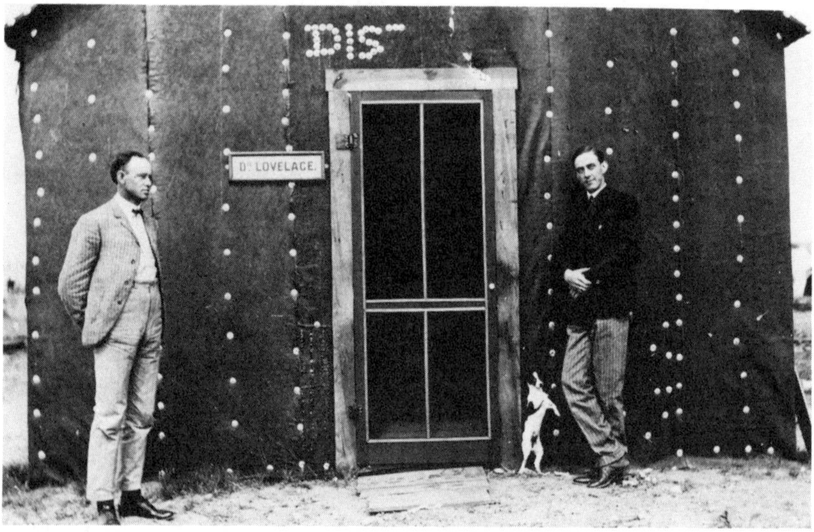

Dr. Lovelace's initial office in Sunnyside (Fort Sumner), New Mexico, was this tarpaper shack supplied by the Santa Fe railroad.

nership with a young pharmacist and his wife.[12] Much of the trauma work associated with railroad mishaps or treatment following the occasional gunfight in town was done in these offices, but the bulk of the country doctor's practice was literally out in the country. Delivering a baby for a sheepherder's wife down on the Maxwell ranch; taking care of the Labadie children in Taiban during a scarlet fever epidemic; setting the leg of a ranchhand injured while tending cattle by Puerta de Luna—such was the standard practice of the frontier doctor. It was work varied enough to challenge the knowledge, skills, and self-confidence of the most experienced doctors. Most of all, perhaps, it challenged the nerves and spirit.

Three specific vignettes remain to us from Dr. Lovelace's Fort Sumner practice. Each illustrates, in different ways, the

12. For a charming account of Dr. Lovelace's practice in Fort Sumner, see "Sutures and Sixguns," *Forum Magazine* (of the Lovelace-Bataan Medical Center) 1, no. 2 (1974): 1–4. This narrative is based on the recollections of Mrs. Lewis Rodrick of Albuquerque, eighty-eight years old at the time of her interview. She was the wife of Dr. Lovelace's pharmacist partner.

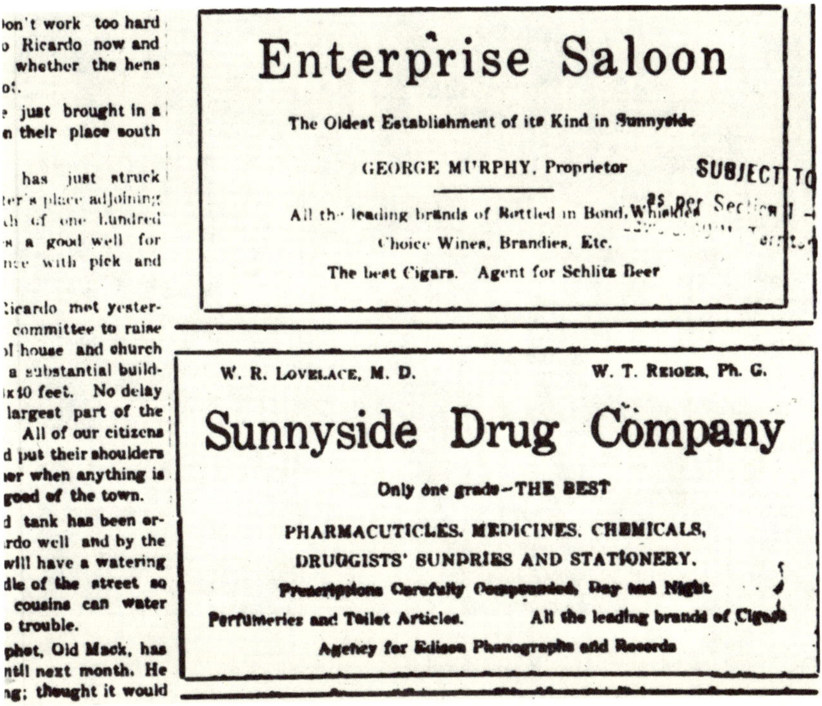

An advertisement from the 9 March 1909 edition of the *Sunnyside Republican,* boosting the drugstore coowned by Dr. Lovelace. Presumably the "pharmacuticles" (sic) available were better than the spelling.

constant challenge faced by the solo practitioner on the raw frontier, far from the relative amenities of medical practice in the cities and towns. For example, the handwritten memoirs of a Fort Sumner woman from the first decades of this century provide some insight into the work of young Dr. Lovelace:

> When he arrived in Sunnyside, he found the conditions usual in a railroad camptown—no accommodations or conveniences of any sort. He had been there a very short while when he was called upon to perform a very delicate operation. A two-year-old boy, son of Isaac Sandoval, a ranch man, was kicked in the head by a shod horse, crushing the skull. The child was brought into town by team, taking two hours for them to make the trip from the

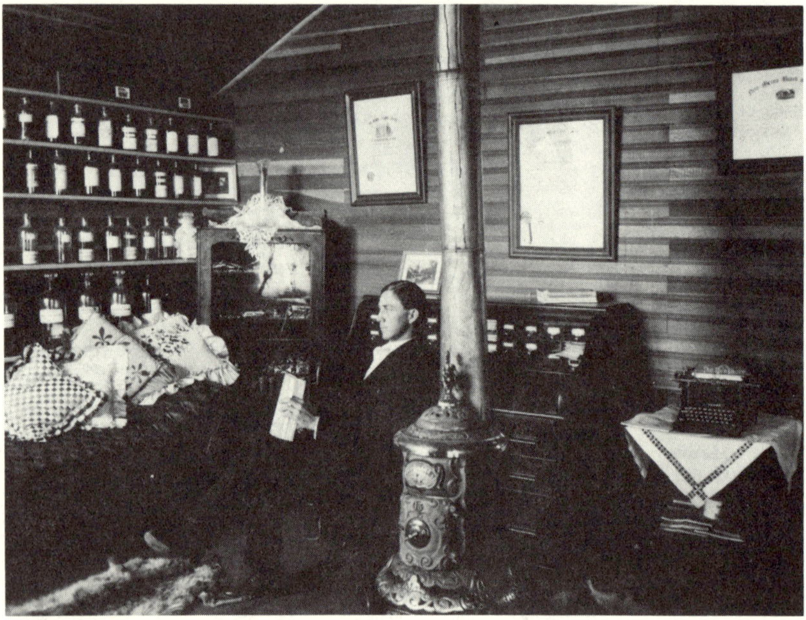

Dr. Lovelace in his neatly organized Fort Sumner office around 1910. Country doctors such as he customarily dispensed their own medicines, hence the rows of medicaments on his wall.

> ranch. His only assistant was one of the Santa Fe nurses stationed there, and by the light of a kerosene lamp he performed this most delicate operation. The boy has grown up to manhood and now resides at Clovis.[13]

More challenging still were the major surgeries performed in the countryside on kitchen tables or crude makeshift operating tables set up in barns. The same source described one such procedure:

> Dr. Lovelace had many miles to ride horseback or drive by team to make sick calls. It was while driving to make one

13. Luisa Beaubien Barrett, "Memoirs," manuscript, Maxwell Land Grant Papers, Special Collections Department, Zimmerman Library, University of New Mexico. The quotation concerning Dr. Lovelace is also contained in a letter held in the Lovelace archives: Clarissa Parsons Fuller, Albuquerque, to Dr. William Randolph Lovelace I, 7 February 1966.

> of his calls to a ranch somewhere the other side of Melrose one evening, a young man met him out in the road and asked him to stop to see his sister who was very ill. Doctor Lovelace told him he'd stop on his way back, as he was on a hurry-up call and couldn't stop, but the young man insisted that he must stop as his sister was dangerously ill and had been alone at their homestead all day. He had found her thus as he came home in the late afternoon. So the doctor stopped at the house and found the young woman in a serious condition. She had received a scratch on her hand with a barbed wire and blood poisoning had set in. Well, he couldn't leave her in that condition and her brother couldn't take her anywhere, as all they had was a team of mules and a wagon, so there was just one thing to do to save the girl's life, and that was to amputate her hand, which he did and the young lady recovered very nicely.[14]

The insistent brother, who would not let the doctor pass by, may have reminded Dr. Lovelace of his very first case in Sunnyside, which came the morning after his arrival from St. Louis and immediately cast the medical (and social) problems of frontier practice in sharp focus for him:

> Along about six the next morning I received my first call. It was to a ranch twelve to fifteen miles below Sunnyside. A boy came up on horseback and said his sister was very sick and I had to come right away. I rented a team and buggy and went with him. Soon after arriving, I examined this eighteen year old girl, then asked her parents, "Is she married?" and they said, "No." I took out my stethoscope and listened for fetal heart sounds and then I knew she was pregnant. She was unconscious and having convulsions, and I took her father outside and said, "I am sorry, but your daughter is pregnant and is going to have a baby. She is having convulsions and we should induce labor. We will have to do something." He said, "Listen, doctor, I want to tell you something. You are a new man out here, and my daughter may be pregnant. But if she is, all right, but if I ever hear of you mentioning it to anyone,

14. Barrett, "Memoirs."

> I will kill you." I said, "Don't you worry, I'll take your word for that. I won't mention it." Well, I thought before leaving I'd try to do something anyway, so I said, "I must examine her closely," then slipped a little instrument between my fingers and ruptured the membranes to induce labor. Immediately after this was done, I got back in the buggy and started to town. The next morning her brother came and said, "Well, we want you to come on back and see my sister. She seems better but not completely conscious." I said, "All right." I returned to the ranch to see her and upon examination found her abdomen was flat and soft. She had delivered the baby, but this fact was not mentioned.[15]

While learning his profession in Fort Sumner and its environs, the neophyte doctor earned the trust and deep affection of the residents of the region. One old-timer waggishly compared his reputation to that of Billy the Kid, claiming that the "kid doctor" was as fast and famous with the knife as the outlaw with his gun.[16] Another recalled:

> His wonderful personality, his ever ready willingness to help everyone, his kindness to rich and poor made him revered. The people of this section of the country learned to love him as their benefactor, and the Spanish-speaking people used to say "Despues de Dios, el Doctor," and he meant just that to them.[17]

In addition to his compassion, his good sense and solidity as a physician and as a person impressed his friends in the Pecos Valley. One of them recommended him in 1909 to Territorial Governor George Curry, with the result that the twenty-six-year-old country doctor was appointed to the five-member New Mexico Board of Medical Examiners, an important governmental agency charged with issuing licenses to practice medicine

15. Lovelace Medical Foundation, Board of Trustees, Minutes, 25 September 1947.

16. Barrett, "Memoirs."

17. "Memorial," author unknown, n.d. (December 1968) in William Randolph Lovelace I files, Lovelace Medical Center Archives.

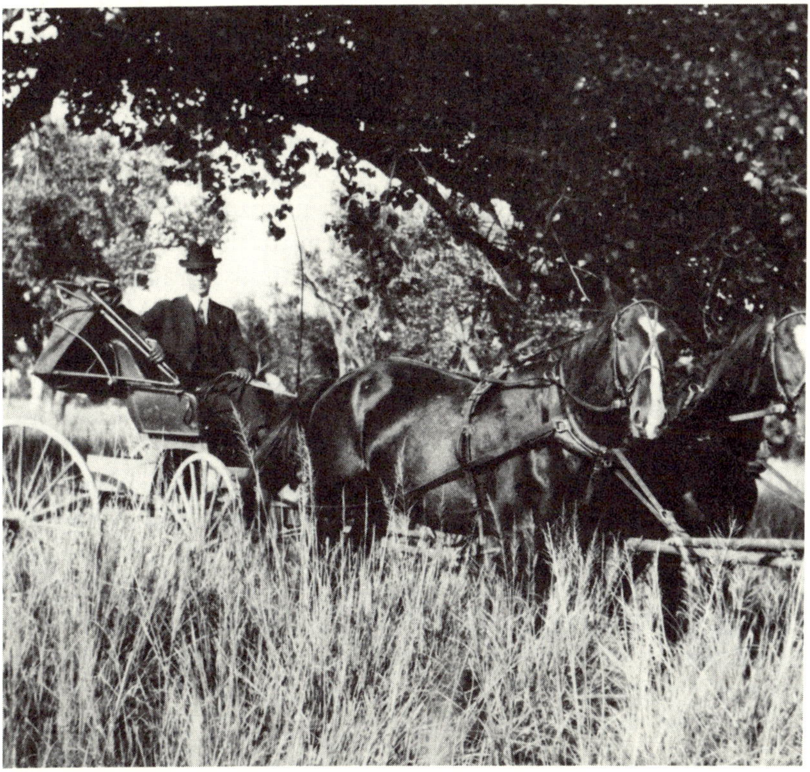

Dr. Lovelace in Fort Sumner, around 1910. He spent much time making calls on horseback or in his buggy, not always so nattily attired as here.

and with general oversight of the profession in the territory. It was a signal honor accorded a young doctor still so new to the region.[18]

His success as a country doctor was complete and undoubtedly satisfying to Dr. Lovelace, but he was not ultimately content with it, however rewarding and important the work might be. He was a markedly ambitious man, interested in a stage larger than the Pecos Valley, and his first years of practice rein-

18. A. P. Anaya, Sunnyside, to Governor George Curry, 5 January 1909, New Mexico Territorial Archives, reel 168, frame 0060. Dr. Lovelace served on the board for twenty-one of the next thirty-eight years, and was its president from 1927–1930.

forced his conviction that he could compete at any level in the medical arena. His ambition and special turn-of-the-century belief in self-help and "drive" were reflected in an advertisement he created for his drugstore in the weekly *Fort Sumner Review:* "We are living in a rapid age—an age of progression. The world moves and you must move with it. If you see a chance to benefit yourself, grasp the opportunity!"[19] But how—and where—to move forward? A return to his native Midwest seemed unrealistic, for he worried about the fragility of his health and the threat to it that a return to the humid Mississippi River Valley would entail. However, Albuquerque, 150 miles to the west, interested him, since its climate was so similar to that of the Pecos Valley and because it was so clearly an enterprising and growing town.

By the time New Mexico became a state in 1912, Albuquerque had overtaken Santa Fe and Las Vegas to become the new state's largest city with 11,020 residents in the official 1910 census. As a railroad and commercial center, its economy was growing rapidly, and it had already established a considerable reputation as an important center of the Southwest's booming tuberculosis industry. Forty years after the fact, Dr. Lovelace remembered the decision to move to Albuquerque:

> All the time I was practicing in Sunnyside, I was thinking about coming to Albuquerque when I had accumulated sufficient money to rent and equip an office. In 1913 I moved to Albuquerque and bought a house for my mother and sisters at 402 Walter and opened an office at 313½ West Central, over the Kistler and Collister Drygoods Store. At the time I left Fort Sumner I had saved $10,000 and bought my first car. After equipping my office, buying the house and car, there was $1,000 left.[20]

19. The ad concluded, "You can benefit yourself by calling on us for anything in the line of Pure Drugs, Chemicals, Standard Patent Medicines, Fancy Goods, Toilet Articles, Perfumery, Stationery and Cigars. Fort Sumner Drug Co." *Fort Sumner Review,* 16 December 1911, p. 2.

20. Lovelace Medical Foundation, Board of Trustees, Minutes, 25 September 1947. The accumulation of 10,000 dollars in savings in seven years of practice in Fort Sumner testifies to the young physician's energies as a physician and to his prudence and ability in managing his money. All who ever knew him—friends and foes alike—testified to his abilities as a businessman.

There was considerable risk associated with the move to Albuquerque. He was solidly established in Fort Sumner country and, indeed, was earning a quite respectable living. In moving to the larger town, he was surrendering that security for the far more competitive Albuquerque marketplace. In Fort Sumner he had been the only doctor in town and one of just a handful patrolling a broad swath of the state's eastern plains. Albuquerque, by contrast, was dangerously overloaded with doctors, for the city's 11,000-plus inhabitants were served by no fewer than 51 physicians, with a physician-to-patient ratio of approximately 1 to 215.[21] However, not all of those doctors were in full, active practice. Some of them lay in the city's sanatoria, of which there were more than a dozen; tuberculars, like Dr. Lovelace, they had come to the city to regain their health. (Many did, but others did not.) Among the city's four dozen physicians also were some retirees and semiretirees, whose practices were tiny or nonexistent. Still there were at least thirty-five busy competitors working in Albuquerque and the area surrounding it; and on balance, they were a highly skilled, reputable crew. Doctors such as P. G. Cornish, Sr., Jacob Easterday, John Elder, Walter G. Hope, Charles Lukens, George McLandress, Eligio Osuna, John Pearce, John Reidy, Lucien G. Rice, Sr., James Wroth, and Meldrum Wylder were already well established in the city—some for more than two decades—and they were men of solid training and commendable skills. No newcomer was going to take Albuquerque by storm. Despite the growing population, it was certain to be a challenge for a new doctor to get established.

Under those circumstances, the rapidity and apparent ease with which twenty-nine-year-old Doctor Lovelace made his way in Albuquerque were remarkable. (From 1911 to 1915, twenty-eight other new physicians tried to set up practice in the town, but only seven of them remained as long as five years.) It is possible that Dr. Lovelace already had something of a modest reputation to precede him. His tenure in Fort Sumner may have made his name familiar to some in Albuquerque, and his appointment to the Board of Medical Examiners in 1912 probably

21. For purposes of comparison, Bernalillo County was generally considered to be oversupplied with physicians in 1985 when its ratio was 1 to 372.

brought him to the attention of other physicians in the town. He quickly secured an appointment as a railroad surgeon with the Santa Fe, presumably by using contacts established during his Fort Sumner connection with the railroad. That linkage brought him some patients and also put him in close contact with many of the community's established doctors through shoulder-to-shoulder work at the sixty-bed Santa Fe Hospital of South Broadway. More important still were the good relations he struck with the Sisters of Charity, who owned and operated St. Joseph Hospital and Sanatorium, a ninety-five-bed general hospital with a forty-bed annex for tuberculosis patients. The close relationship with the Sisters was one of the cornerstones of Dr. Lovelace's success in Albuquerque. He was an especially important figure in the hospital's energetic expansion in the 1920s and 1930s, working as a near partner of the administration during the tenures of Sister Philip Neri and, later, Sister Mary Lawrence as St. Joseph Hospital Administrator. (The charge was sometimes made in the 1930s and 1940s that Dr. Lovelace "controlled" St. Joseph hospital.) Most of his practice was focused in St. Joseph and the Santa Fe hospitals, but he was also appointed to the staffs of the Southwestern Presbyterian Sanatorium and the Methodist Sanatorium, both located on East Central Avenue (then called "San Alley"). His quick, full acceptance by the Albuquerque medical establishment was capped in December 1915 by his election as president of the Bernalillo County Medical Association for the year of 1916. Few other physicians were able to crack the Albuquerque establishment so quickly and decisively.

Two major developments marked Dr. Lovelace's first decade in Albuquerque. In 1915, the ambitious young surgeon made the first of many trips to that lodestar of American medicine, the Mayo Clinic in Rochester, Minnesota. Of course, he was only one among many attracted to that midwestern medical center by its reputation for excellence and its progressive approach to the practice of medicine. Did he first go to Mayo, as many did, as part of a continuing educational process to sharpen his surgical skills? Or was he more particularly interested in the way that the Mayo brothers had organized their flagship clinic? Group practice on the Mayo model was still unusual in

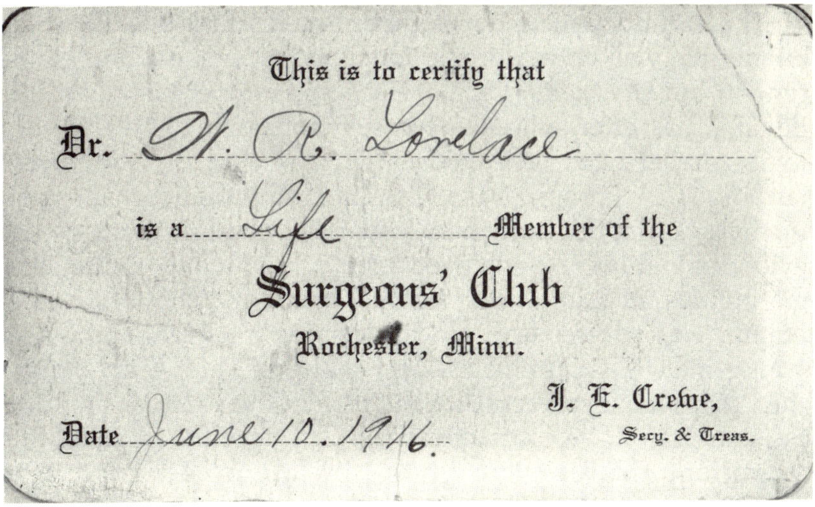

This is to certify that

Dr. W. R. Lovelace

is a Life Member of the

Surgeons' Club

Rochester, Minn.

J. E. Crewe,
Secy. & Treas.

Date June 10. 1916.

Dr. Lovelace to the end of his long life was proud of his life membership in the Mayo Clinic's Surgeon's Club.

the 1910s, for the very great majority of American practitioners were still firmly wed to the tradition of solo practice, in which every man was a free agent unto himself. Whatever his motivation—and it was probably a little of each—he was captivated by what he saw in Rochester. In his estimation, the Mayo operation was clearly the way of the future, the model for the modern, efficient, twentieth-century practice of medicine. He was also inspired by personal contact with the brothers Mayo themselves, Drs. Will and Charlie, and developed a lifelong personal friendship with them. To his last days, he was very proud of the fact that he had become a life member of the Mayo Surgeons' Club as early as 1916.[22] From the time of that very first visit in 1915, it was his ambition to transplant the Mayo system—or at least as much of it as he could manage—to the far Southwest, to set up a modern medical center modeled after the Rochester institution.

22. There is evidence that Dr. Lovelace often stayed in the home of Dr. Will Mayo on his trips to Rochester, but a far stronger personal relationship was forged within the next generation between the senior Dr. Lovelace's nephew, Dr. Randy Lovelace, and Dr. Charles W. Mayo, son of founder Dr. Will Mayo.

The second critical development of his first decade in Albuquerque was both a professional and a personal one. Some time in the late teens, Dr. Lovelace met a quiet Georgian, Dr. Edgar T. Lassetter, who, like himself, had come to New Mexico to seek relief from tuberculosis. Dr. Lassetter, too, was from farming stock, although his Georgia family was perhaps a cut up the social ladder from the Missouri Lovelaces. (There is some evidence that his father played a fairly prominent role in Georgia politics, at least at the regional level, and the loftier term planter was sometimes used to describe his livelihood.) As a young man, Ed Lassetter served with the U.S. Army during the Philippine insurrection at the turn of the century; and during that period, he contracted the pulmonary tuberculosis that later prompted his migration to New Mexico Territory. After military service, he returned to his native Georgia and earned a pharmacy degree from Atlanta's Southern College of Pharmacy in 1907. A short period of practice as a pharmacist in his native Butts County was ended in early 1909, however, by serious deterioration of his lung condition, and the thirty-five-year-old Lassetter was forced to seek recovery of his health in the more salubrious high country of the Southwest.

As a military veteran, Lassetter was eligible for treatment at the United States Army General Hospital in Fort Bayard, New Mexico. That institution—a large four-hundred-bed facility opened in 1899 and used almost exclusively as a tuberculosis sanatorium—had on its staff several of the most highly respected tuberculosis specialists in the nation, including Drs. George E. Bushnell and Earl S. Bullock. They successfully directed the Georgian's treatment, and influenced his career ambitions as well. During nearly three years of convalescence at Fort Bayard, Lassetter not only recovered his health, but also was powerfully affected by the example of the devoted doctors who supervised his care. He determined to shift from pharmacy to medicine and, though he was fast approaching forty, he entered the Southern College of Medicine and Surgery upon his return to Georgia in late 1911 or 1912.

The question of Dr. Lassetter's formal medical education requires some specific discussion, for in later years opponents of the Lovelace Clinic (of which Dr. Lassetter was a full partner) made aspersions regarding the supposed weakness of his med-

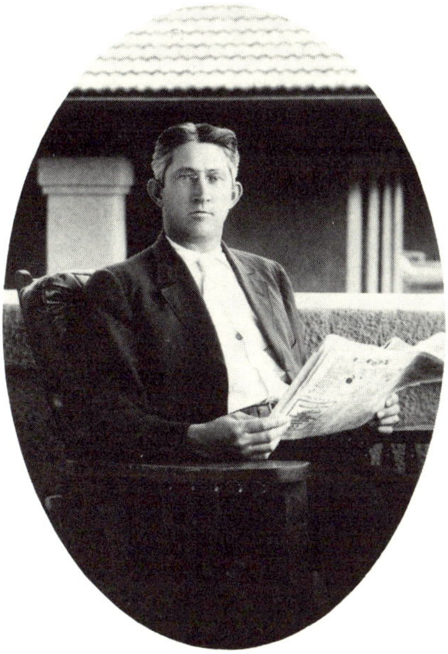

Dr. Edgar T. Lassetter in Fort Bayard, 1914.

ical credentials. Apparently, he started his medical schooling at the Atlanta School of Medicine, a proprietary institution first opened in 1905, and then finished his formal studies at Southern College of Medicine and Surgery, newly opened in 1911. Both these institutions were ephemeral and of minimal quality, hardly deserving the label "medical school." That reality alone made the solidity of Lassetter's formal preparation at least questionable. In addition, the exact tenure of Ed Lassetter's study in those schools is uncertain; it may have been as little as eighteen months, possibly even less. (Presumably, he would have received some kind of credit for his work toward a pharmacy degree.) Clearly, the quality of his medical education was open to question, although questions were never raised about his capabilities and genuine gifts as a practicing physician.[23] Ad-

23. Somewhere or other—if not at the shaky Atlanta medical schools he attended—Ed Lassetter learned a great deal about medicine and the medical sciences. When he applied for medical licensure in New Mexico in the spring of 1914, he was required to take the formal qualifying examination of the state's Board of Medical Examiners. He scored 90 percent or higher in bacteriology, physiology, surgery, hygiene, practice of medicine, and physical diagnosis, and comfortably passed everything else, too. Board of Medical Examiners, Minutes, 13 April and 13 July 1914.

versaries of the Lovelace Clinic, however, raised the question often, referring to the "education problem" in their criticism of the Lovelace-Lassetter partnership. The subject was thoroughly, if discreetly, discussed within Albuquerque medical circles. Incidentally, it is highly probable that the questions raised about the quality of Dr. *Lovelace's* medical education (see n.3, above) actually originated in the gossip—confused in the telling—regarding Dr. *Lassetter's* formal medical studies. Dr. Lassetter himself was apparently aware of these questions, which ultimately brought into doubt his "legitimacy" as a physician. They were probably the major factor in his decision not to apply for membership in the Bernalillo County Medical Association, the bastion of the "regular" physicians in Albuquerque, until more than twenty years after his arrival. Even then, although his abilities as a physician were absolutely proven, the old issue of his education haunted him. When he did finally apply (for whatever reason) in January 1935, there was much discreet parliamentary maneuvering not fully spelled out in the society's minutes, with the result that discussion and a vote on his application were postponed. Before the next meeting, Dr. Lassetter apparently withdrew his name from consideration.[24]

After completing his controversial Atlanta schooling in May 1913, Dr. Lassetter returned to New Mexico, again to Fort Bayard. Perhaps his health was still threatened, and he chose to return to that part of the country which had done so much to improve his condition five years earlier. In Fort Bayard, while continuing his cure, he practiced medicine on at least a part-time basis. This time his recovery was complete, and in 1918 he was strong enough to move to Albuquerque to try to establish himself in private practice. Like Dr. Lovelace five years earlier, Ed Lassetter was able to survive and then thrive in the competitive world of Albuquerque medicine. It was quickly evident that he had a special gift for diagnosis—which remained his strong suit throughout the thirty-plus years of his practice—and that he possessed the special compassion and

24. Bernalillo County Medical Association, Minutes, 8 January and 7 February 1935.

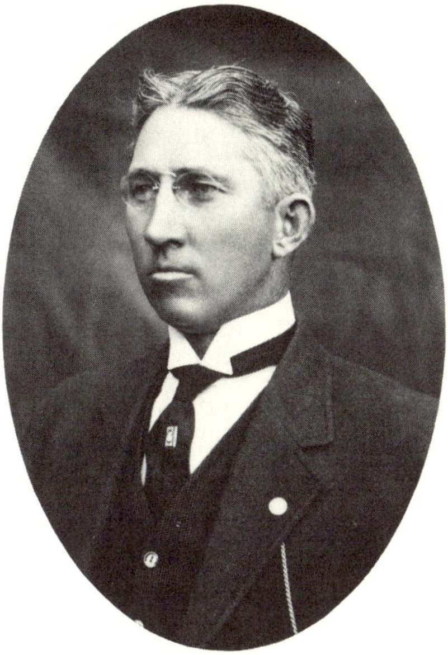

Dr. Lassetter in a formal portrait dating from the late 1910s.

dedication associated with the best among the old-time country doctors and general practitioners. He was devoted to his patients and both Drs. Lovelace and Lassetter became legendary for their attentiveness to their patients. Throughout almost all of their active medical careers, they worked without the supporting array of sophisticated medicines and the modern diagnostic and therapeutic equipment and technical aids available to modern physicians; but what they had—their learning, experience, time, and sympathetic ears—they gave unstintingly to the ailing men and women who turned to them for help.

Soon after his relocation to Albuquerque, Dr. Lassetter met the already established Dr. Lovelace through the latter's younger sister Lora. The two physicians quickly found that they had much in common. For example, each was animated by an intense commitment to his profession; both possessed the strong conviction that the life of a physician was a "calling" in an almost religious sense; each organized his practice (and his life) on the unwavering principle that the patient and his or her needs always came first; and both men were confident that hard work and fair dealing would earn both honor and (not to be ignored) a solid, comfortable livelihood. On these principles Drs. Lovelace and Lassetter forged firm professional ties, and their linkage was cemented by a personal one as well, when Dr. Lassetter married Lora Lovelace in 1919. For the three decades that followed—until Dr. Lassetter's death in 1948—Drs. Lovelace and Lassetter were a closely knit professional and personal team. There is no record that any serious professional or personal disagreement or discord ruffled the smoothness of the relationship. Professionally, their cooperation was facilitated by the complementarity of their individual skills and interests. Both were general practitioners throughout the 1920s and 1930s, but Dr. Lovelace increasingly developed a special interest and competency in surgery, while Dr. Lassetter tilted his practice in the direction of what would today be called internal medicine. At the personal level, their basic values were similar and their personalities meshed neatly. Dr. Lovelace was distinctly the more aggressive of the two—restless, energetic, and fiercely ambitious. Dr. Lassetter was much quieter, even retiring, and entirely content to let his brother-in-law take the leadership role in the relationship. For his part, Dr. Lovelace was unfailingly respectful of his partner and always evinced the most profound regard for him. Although Dr. Lovelace was the active, driving force within the tandem, he always honored the wisdom, hard work, and good judgment of Dr. Lassetter. For example, it was Dr. Lovelace in the 1950s who insisted that one of the first major research facilities erected by the Lovelace Foundation for Medical Education and Research be named after his late partner.

The two doctors began to merge their practices in 1919, initially sharing Dr. Lovelace's offices at 313½ West Central Avenue over the Kistler-Collister store. (They also lived in adjacent houses further out West Central Avenue.) It was not until 1922, however, that their association became a formal partnership. At first, the straightforward label "Lovelace and Lassetter" identified the partnership, but by the end of the 1920s the new designation "Lovelace Clinic" was in use. (There is no record of its use before 1929.) Nevertheless, 1922 is conventionally cited in all of the institution's documents as the birth-year of the Lovelace Clinic.[25] Thus, from the anxious flight to New Mexico Territory of two "lunger" physicians was born an institution that was to have a profound impact on health care in the Southwest.

25. Dr. Lovelace himself always regarded it that way. See his personal sketch of his own and the clinic's history in Lovelace Medical Foundation, Board of Trustees, Minutes, 25 September 1947.

TWO

The Clinic's Early Years

In the quarter-century between the founding of the Lovelace Clinic in 1922 and its radical transformation in 1947, the simple institution created by Drs. Lovelace and Lassetter became a prominent force in Albuquerque and in New Mexico medicine. In building on the foundation of the founders' personal practices and gradually expanding from it, the Lovelace Clinic rapidly developed a tradition of excellence and innovation. Simultaneously, it became one party to a frequently bitter professional split within the Albuquerque medical community, a division which was to be a pronounced feature of the region's medical culture for almost half a century. To some degree, the split was a function of Dr. Lovelace's fierce competitiveness and sometimes brusque manner; but even more, it was the product of the decision made by Drs. Lovelace and Lassetter in the late 1920s to expand their successful partnership into the Southwest's first group practice.

Although the Lovelace Clinic was born in three small rooms over a dry-goods store, it quickly took on a more modern and fashionable face when it moved in late 1923 to the new First National Bank building at the corner of Third and Central in downtown Albuquerque. Like many of the "better" doctors in town, Drs. Lovelace and Lassetter immediately moved into the new structure, occupying rooms 304, 305, 306, 307, and 308 on the third floor and answering telephone number 985. The immediate and wholesale migration of doctors to the new office building reflected its choice location. The bank building sat

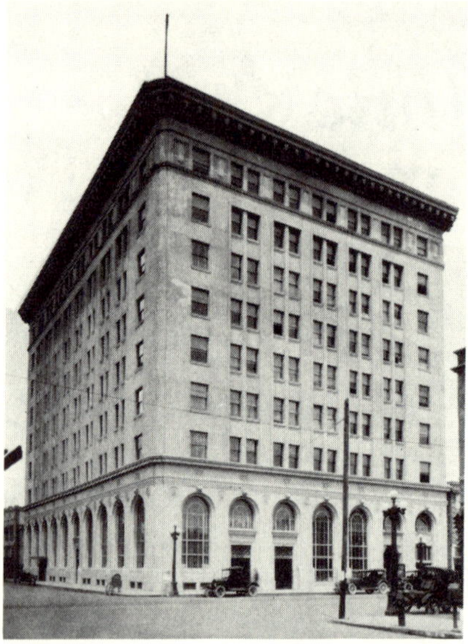

The First National Bank building in downtown Albuquerque, initial site of the Lovelace Clinic from 1923 to 1950.

astride old Route 66, piercing the city east to west, and it was within a couple of blocks of both the Santa Fe railroad line and Federal Highway 85, running from Santa Fe and points north down the Rio Grande Valley to El Paso. Convenient to all of the town's hospitals, it was right at the heart of downtown Albuquerque, which was then still the commercial, governmental, and professional hub of the city. Within a few months of its opening, the bank building was host to no fewer than twenty-five MDs and one osteopath—roughly half the city's total complement of actively practicing physicians. The partnership of Lovelace and Lassetter did not stand out at first within that constellation of doctors, even though it occupied a full five rooms on the building's third floor. Several of the solo practitioners—at least the busier doctors among them—rented three- or four-room offices; but as time passed and the Lovelace Clinic prospered, the clinic came to occupy the entire floor. (In the late 1940s, it even spilled over into an adjacent building to the north.) For nearly thirty years, the Lovelace Clinic was identified with the downtown bank building. It was only with the redefinition of its mission in 1947 that new physical facilities became absolutely necessary.

After the formation of the Lovelace-Lassetter partnership in 1922 and the move into the bank building the next year, the remainder of the decade was a period of quiet, unspectacular growth for the enterprise. During that time, for example, Dr. Lovelace expanded his already substantial surgical practice into one of the largest in the Southwest. He developed a particular interest in surgical treatment of tuberculosis—in a time when large numbers of tuberculars were still flowing into the region—and worked hard to stay abreast of the latest approaches to dealing with the disease. In 1923, for instance, he played host to an eminent Canadian surgeon, Dr. John Archibald of Toronto, and from him Lovelace learned to do thoracoplasties for the relief of selected tuberculosis cases. Periodically, the ever-learning and growing Albuquerque surgeon took the time to write up case reports from his practice, publishing them in reputable professional journals, including the *Journal of the American Medical Association.*[1] It seems clear that he never developed the surgical skills and range that would have ranked him among the recognized leaders of the field, but as a largely self-taught "country surgeon," he fashioned a commendable record, one of which he was justifiably proud. His almost annual trips to the Mayo Clinic and to other American surgical centers were intended fundamentally to keep him up to date with developments in surgery and to hone his own skills. In the 1930s he began to supplement those trips with study tours to major European surgical centers and such diligence paid off in increasing stature among his peers. Seen in his proper geographic and chronological context, he established a commendable record as a general surgeon and commanded widespread respect within the Southwest.

While constructing his large general surgery practice and

1. William R. Lovelace, Walter A. Gekler, H. P. Rankin, and V. J. Weigel, "Tuberculous Cavitation of the Lung: Mechanical Factors in Its Genesis and Combined Chemotherapeutic and Surgical Treatment," *JAMA* 82 (1924):457–63; and William R. Lovelace, "Fibrolipoma of Left Labium Majora," *JAMA* 80 (1923):375–77. Two other samples from his bibliography of the 1920s and 1930s are "The Surgical Treatment of Tuberculosis" *Southwestern Medicine* 10 (1926):472–77, and "Implantation of a Biliary Fistula into the Gastrointestinal Tract: Case Report and Two Year Follow-Up," *Southwestern Medicine* 16 (1932):159–64.

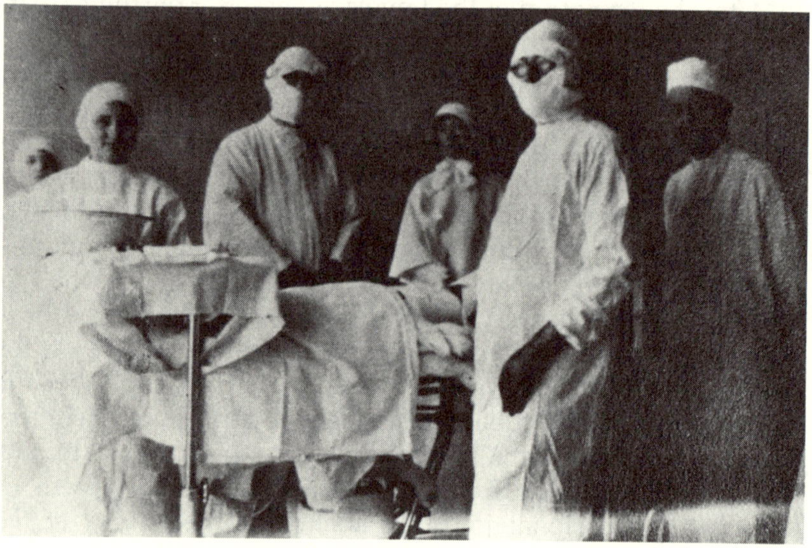

Drs. Lovelace and Lassetter in the operating room at St. Joseph Hospital sometime in the 1920s. Dr. Lovelace is in the center foreground of the picture, and Dr. Lassetter is on the opposite side of the table.

working conscientiously to expand and improve his skills, Dr. Lovelace also found time for extensive involvement with his family and for making an impressive personal fortune through prudent real estate investment. Although he never married—supposedly, he left a grieving fiancée back in Missouri when be broke down with tuberculosis, and had many interesting, attractive lady friends throughout his life—he invested much of his time and psychic energies in the affairs of his extended family. Within the domestic sphere he was clearly paterfamilias, caring for and directing not only his own broad-range personal affairs, but also, to a large degree, those of his parents and siblings.[2] His parents and his much-beloved two younger sisters all lived under his roof for extended periods of time, and his

2. The best source for details of the Lovelace family history is Richard G. Elliott, " 'On a Comet, Always.' A Biography of William Randolph Lovelace II," *New Mexico Quarterly* 36, no. 4 (1966–67):351–88. I am grateful to Mr. Elliott for generously sharing his materials and perspectives with me during the writing of this book.

older brother was also disposed to accept his leadership. Both of his parents lived with him until their deaths in the 1940s, and after the collapse of her marriage, his sister Maybelle Westerfield shared his home during the last four decades of her life, serving as his hostess. Younger sister Lora, who had married Dr. Lassetter, was never very far away, and she returned to the large Lovelace family home on North Twelfth Street in downtown Albuquerque after her husband's death in 1948. Clearly the bachelor surgeon enjoyed a full family life, and his influence as head of the family extended powerfully into the next generation as well.

One of the family relationships controlled by Dr. Lovelace proved to be of cardinal significance in the long-term development of the Lovelace Clinic. In 1908, older brother Edgar Lovelace, with his wife and six-month-old son William Randolph Lovelace II, or Randy, had joined the rest of the family in New Mexico. Randy Lovelace was the eldest of three nephews whose upbringing, education, and career choices were heavily influenced, if not simply controlled, by their uncle.[3] During his boyhood and adolescence, Randy spent considerable time with his grandmother and "Uncle Doc"[4] at the latter's downtown Albuquerque home. After the divorce of his parents in 1918, the eleven-year-old boy moved from his father's ranch near Gran Quivira, New Mexico, to Albuquerque to live with his uncle and grandmother. For the seven years of his adolescence, then, prior to leaving to attend college in 1925, Randy Lovelace was under the direct supervision of his Uncle Doc.

3. The second eldest nephew was Maybelle Lovelace Westerfield's son Frank, who became an attorney prominent in Albuquerque legal circles. The youngest was Edgar Lovelace Lassetter, son of Dr. Edgar T. and Lora Lovelace Lassetter. Eddie Lassetter became a physician like his father and uncle before him, and he was on the staff of the Lovelace Clinic from 1951 until his retirement in 1982.

4. Something should be said regarding this nickname conventionally applied to the senior Dr. Lovelace, or William Randolph Lovelace I (hereafter cited as WRL I). Since Randy (hereafter cited as WRL II) also became a physician, "Uncle Doc" was a label of convenience that was useful in differentiating between the two. It was not so much a term of affection, for WRL I was never a particularly approachable man. In his maturity, he was a somewhat austere, even forbidding figure who commanded respect, but not necessarily affection—except among his patients! Incidentally, he himself accepted and used the nickname "Uncle Doc" in signing personal and family correspondence.

More will be said later of Randy Lovelace, his close relationship to his demanding uncle, and his role in the creation and development of the Lovelace Foundation for Medical Education and Research. He is mentioned here to suggest the full range and variety of family responsibilities carried by the senior Dr. Lovelace in the twenties and thirties, while he was planning and preparing for the more ambitious professional ventures yet to come.

During the era between wars, he began to earn a significant amount of money and to invest it wisely for the future. His physician's charges were modest, entirely consistent with the prevailing Albuquerque rates, but his practice simply became so large that considerable sums came in via the late-night house calls, the surgeries, and the regular office schedule of the active physician. More importantly, he husbanded his money wisely, and the income from his investments soon rivaled and then surpassed that of his profitable practice. Financially conservative, he invested mostly in land and in safe government bonds. By the time of the Second World War, he had become one of the most important land owners in Albuquerque. He was no land "speculator" in the sense of buying and selling parcels of land in the hope of quick returns on his money. Rather, he bought and kept what he thought to be good parcels of land that were likely to appreciate significantly over time. Both commercial property in downtown Albuquerque and vacant land on the city's east mesa attracted his attention.[5] Early on, he developed the policy of deciding for himself what, when, and where to buy, and throughout fifty years of land trading in

5. His most valuable piece of downtown property was the land at the northwest corner of Fifth and Central, on which he erected the building which he rented to Sears, Roebuck as the site of its main retail outlet in Albuquerque; but he also owned large parcels of land on Fourth Street, both north and south of Central Avenue. In the residential sections of the town, he concentrated his holdings in what are now the northeast and southeast heights of the metropolitan region. For example, he owned all of the land from the corner of Gibson Boulevard and San Mateo east to Louisiana Boulevard—the property on which the Lovelace Medical Center, Siesta Hills subdivision, and much else presently stands; the land now known as the Hoffmantown addition and the Snow Heights subdivision; large tracts of land near the present-day airport and Yale Boulevard; as well as other properties. He was not interested in land outside Albuquerque, although he did secure various small properties from time to time.

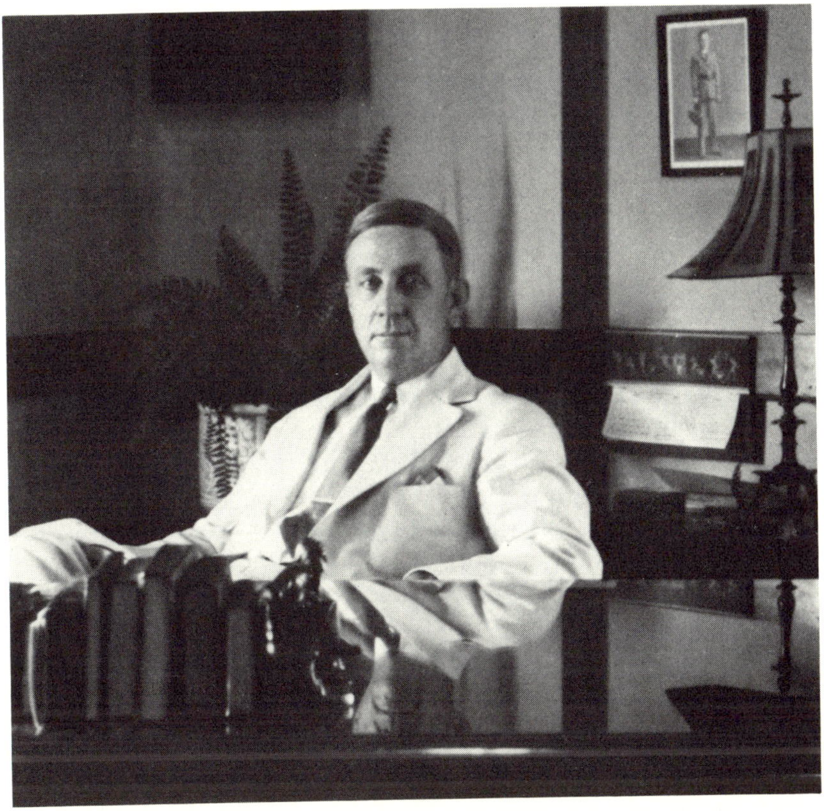

Dr. Lovelace, a portrait from the 1920s.

Albuquerque, he basically trusted to his own instincts and judgments.[6] As a result, he accumulated a sizeable personal fortune rising well into six figures and perhaps higher by the outbreak of the war.

Some of Dr. Lovelace's financial success was attributable to the steady, solid growth of the Albuquerque economy and pop-

6. These remarks on Uncle Doc's real estate ventures are based on an interview with George Savage, a major real estate figure in Albuquerque from the early 1920s until his retirement in the 1970s, and a realtor with whom Uncle Doc frequently worked. George Savage, interview with the author, Albuquerque, New Mexico, 8 February 1985. I also learned much about Uncle Doc as a businessman from John Dornacker, an accountant, stock broker, and longtime friend of the Lovelace family. John Dornacker, interview with the author, Albuquerque, 7 March 1985.

ulation in the twenties and thirties, which almost guaranteed success to a careful land investor. More important, however, was his own hardheaded business sense. Everyone who knew him well particularly respected his capacity for making money.[7] One key element in that talent was his keen sensitivity to the costs of doing things. In his later years, he became legendary at Lovelace Foundation board meetings for his ability to listen politely to a proposal or new program and then penetrate to the heart of the discussion with his standard query, "Where're you going to get the money?" His business and managerial sense was critical to the rise of the Lovelace Clinic from its birth in the twenties until the end of the war, and when circumstances required it, he always put his personal fortune solidly behind the institution. His munificent gifts of land and money to the Lovelace Foundation will be discussed below; here it should be emphasized that Dr. Lovelace's business judgment and consequently, his personal fortune were fundamental elements in the long-term growth and success of the Lovelace Clinic and, later, of the Lovelace Foundation. As late as 1966, when Uncle Doc was eighty-three years old and far removed from the direction of the institution he had created, he could still be counted on to come up with an emergency loan of more than twenty thousand dollars—without interest—to help in resolving a temporary collections shortfall. Although he was known as a "hard man with a dollar," he was consistently and ungrudgingly generous to the medical complex which bore his name.[8]

Sometime in the late 1920s, Drs. Lovelace and Lassetter made a decision that set their busy partnership on a radically new course. They decided to expand their practice from a simple partnership into a group practice, employing other doctors to work for them. And there was to be a particular thrust to

7. Years after the fact, the powerful and successful businessman C. R. Smith, longtime president of American Airlines and secretary of commerce in Richard Nixon's first cabinet, remembered with respect Dr. Lovelace's flair for business: "he sure knew how to make money . . . and how to take care of it, too!" C. R. Smith, interview with the author, Washington, D.C., 7 January 1985.

8. Promissory note, 28 March 1966, in WRL I file, Lovelace Medical Center Archives.

their projected expansion: they would hire trained specialists, modern doctors with particular training and expertise. There is no hard evidence available to trace the logic of that decision, no "memorandum of understanding" or other document in which the partners spelled out their plans for the future and the factors conditioning their thinking.[9] Nevertheless, it is almost certain that their decision to expand, and to do so in a particular way, arose from three interrelated factors.

First, and most immediately important, was the stark reality that the two doctors had more business than they could handle comfortably and badly needed help. The few records available from the 1920s and the ampler indirect evidence plainly indicate that the partnership experienced pronounced growth during that decade. Office hours expanded year by year, but the volume of patient office calls to the bank building swelled commensurately, constantly increasing pressure on the two physicians' office schedules. House calls remained a central part of their practices, but house calls in Albuquerque and its immediate environs were only one part of that aspect of their practice. Doctor Lovelace sometimes rode the train to Fort Sumner to take care of a patient-friend, and in his trusty, "physicianly" Buick he bounced across unpaved roads as far as St. Johns, Arizona, to tend to longtime patients.[10] In addition, Dr. Lovelace maintained his full surgical schedule at St. Joseph Hospital; Dr. Lassetter made his hospital rounds; and both men delivered babies as well as constantly responding to acute illnesses of whatever description. Around the edges of that busy, almost frantic practice, Dr. Lovelace managed to include active participation in professional organizations such as the International College of Surgeons, the Bernalillo County Medical

9. Long after the fact, Uncle Doc discussed his concern "that the field of medicine was changing and expanding so rapidly that it was impossible for any one man to command it," which was, he declared, the major determinant in convincing him that a group practice of thoroughly trained specialists provided the proper organization for the medicine of the future. Lovelace Medical Foundation, Board of Trustees, Minutes, 25 September 1947.

10. Years later, the sister of one of his patients wrote to him, "I first knew you when you graciously drove all the way to St. Johns to help the Lord save the life of my dear brother Albert." Letty A. Patterson, Atlanta, to WRL I, 13 January 1966, in WRL I file, Lovelace Medical Center archives.

Association, the state medical society, the New Mexico Board of Medical Examiners, the city hospital staffs, and many others.

The pressures and demands of their growing practices reminded Drs. Lovelace and Lassetter on a daily basis of the necessity for some modification of their practice style, and it was the inspiring example of the Mayo Clinic that pointed a specific way. Dr. Lovelace had been strongly impressed with the Minnesota institution as early as 1915, and his repeated trips to it during the subsequent fifteen years reinforced his earlier judgment that group practice involving the full spectrum of modern specialization was the most efficient and responsible means of organizing future medical practice. He had been eminently successful as a solo practitioner; but like many other physicians around the country, he was not content that the traditional model of solo practice was best suited to the rapidly changing circumstances of the twentieth century. The birth of the Lovelace Clinic in 1922 made it a phenomenon contemporary with such other prominent group practices as Boston's Lahey Clinic, Seattle's Mason Clinic, the Henry Ford Hospital group practice in Detroit, the Cleveland Clinic, and others. In fact, the 1920s and early 1930s were a time of explosive growth for the American group-practice movement.[11] Albuquerque and the Southwest generally were solid bastions of the individual practitioner, but Lovelace and Lassetter determined to challenge the traditional model.

In at least a marginal way, family considerations or loyalties also helped to encourage thought about group practice. Relatives of both Drs. Lovelace and Lassetter came to practice with the two men in the 1920s, and this association provided some experience in group practice. One such physician-relative who came to Albuquerque and practiced within the Lovelace-Lassetter operation was Dr. Loren Elliott. A general practitioner with a special interest in surgery, Dr. Elliott was a cousin of Dr. Lovelace, a member of the Walker (the maternal) side of his family. The newcomer was ten years younger than his cou-

11. On the birth and development of group practice in this country, see C. Rufus Rorem, *Private Group Clinics* (Chicago: University of Chicago Press, 1931); American Medical Association, Bureau of Medical Economics, *Group Practice* (Chicago: American Medical Association, 1933); and Paul Starr, *The Social Transformation of American Medicine* (New York: Basic Books, 1982), esp. pp. 209–15.

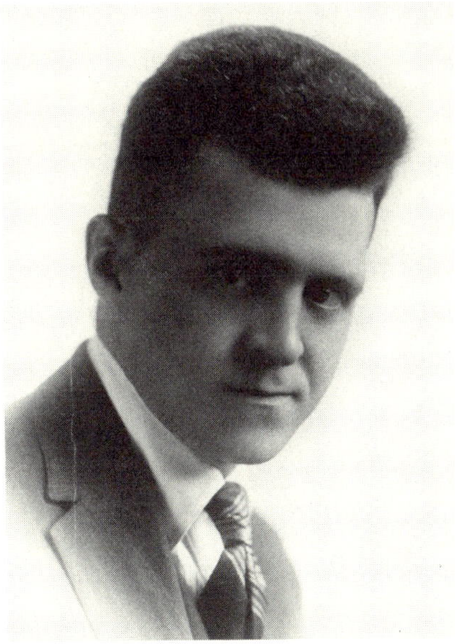

Dr. Loren Elliott, around 1920.

sin, and like Lovelace, he had left the farm country around Rolla, Missouri, to attend the St. Louis University School of Medicine, where he graduated in 1919. In the first half of the 1920s, Elliott interspersed periods of advanced study, mostly in surgery, with practice stints in Albuquerque; and in joining Drs. Lovelace and Lassetter in the bank building, he relieved some of their burden. Then, in 1925, Dr. Elliott moved permanently to Albuquerque, to work for the older men as a salaried physician. Dr. Elliott stayed with the Lovelace and Lassetter partnership for three years; then, for reasons unknown, he left them to set up a private practice in the bank building. He practiced in the Albuquerque community until his death in late 1949. After going into private practice, relations between Dr. Elliott and the older men were not good, and for most of the two decades that followed, Loren Elliott was clearly a member of the anti-Lovelace segment of the Albuquerque medical community.[12]

12. See Loren F. Elliott file, Lovelace Medical Center archives. The apparent breach between Elliott and the Lovelace-Lassetter partners—professional, personal or both? —may help to explain Dr. Lovelace's subsequent rigid insistence on a restrictive covenant clause in the contracts of Lovelace Clinic doctors (see chap. 6, pp. 146–147).

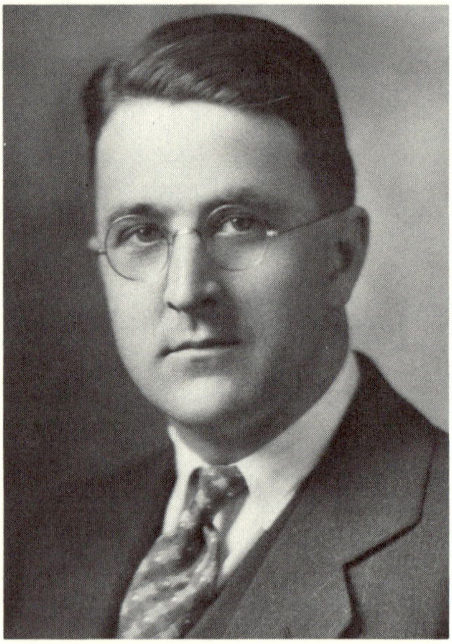

Dr. J. Daniel Lamon, 1929.

Following Dr. Elliott's departure, Dr. John Daniel Lamon joined the Lovelace and Lassetter partnership. Dan Lamon's arrival in Albuquerque in March 1929 marked a kind of Rubicon in the elaboration of the Lovelace Clinic. His employment was the decisive step taken by Drs. Lovelace and Lassetter toward transforming the partnership into a large, multispecialty group practice. Dr. Lamon, a Georgia-born and -reared nephew of Dr. Lassetter, had received his medical degree at the Medical College of Georgia in 1925. After advanced training in general surgery at some of the better surgical centers of the East Coast, including two and a half years at the Reconstructive Polyclinic, and Presbyterian hospitals in New York City, he had capped his preparation at the Mayo Clinic. Lamon, in short, represented the new wave specialist with impressive professional credentials, and was just the kind of candidate with whom to inaugurate the group-practice experiment.

The arrival of Dr. Lamon did more than simply initiate a group practice. It also provoked the first salvos in what became a fifty-year-long war between the Lovelace Clinic and a substantial segment of the other physicians of the Albuquerque medical community, who were usually called the "downtown docs."[13] The first sign of the brewing trouble appeared only three weeks after Dr. Lamon's arrival. The venue of the antagonism was the Bernalillo County Medical Association, and the minutes of that organization succinctly register the discordance:

> The question of recent advertizements which have appeared in the newspapers was brot [sic] up and discussed. Dr. Lovelace stated he desired the matter be thoroly [sic] investigated. Motion by Dr. Lovelace that the chair appoint a committee of three to investigate these recent write-ups as to authenticated sources and report back to the society.[14]

The offending "advertisement" was an innocuous twenty-one-word notice in the "Society" column of the *Albuquerque Journal* of 9 March 1929:

> Dr. Daniel Lamon will arrive on Saturday from Mayo's Clinic. He will be associated with Drs. W. R. Lovelace and E. T. Lassetter.[15]

This first of many disputes between the downtown doctors and the Lovelace Clinic ended quietly enough with a bland committee report that found Dr. Lovelace "blameless for these articles,"[16] but the small tempest was an unpleasant harbinger of many subsequent and similar conflicts.

Without doubt, many physicians of the Albuquerque community were genuinely offended by the "advertising" in what

13. This was the terminology employed after 1950, when the Lovelace Clinic moved from the downtown bank building to its new clinic building in Albuquerque's southeast suburbs. Thereafter, the anti-Lovelace faction was called the "downtown docs" because of their concentration in and around the downtown hospitals; especially Presbyterian Hospital, where they controlled the staff. Dr. Albert G. Simms, interview with the author, Albuquerque, 17 and 18 May 1984 and Dr. P. G. Cornish III, interview with the author, Albuquerque, 21 November 1983; and other interviews.

14. Bernalillo County Medical Association, Minutes, 3 April 1929.

15. *Albuquerque Journal* (evening edition), 9 March 1929. A similar notice ran in the "Town Talk" column of the *New Mexico State Tribune* (Albuquerque), 9 March 1929.

16. Bernalillo County Medical Association, Minutes, 1 May 1929.

now appears to be no more than an innocent announcement of Dr. Lamon's arrival in town. Well into the twentieth century, physicians were expected to avoid scrupulously any mention of their names by newspapers in order to avoid even the slightest hint of hucksterism within the profession. However, on this particular occasion, the keen ire of the downtown doctors resulted not so much from the "advertising" itself, but because Dr. Lamon's arrival meant the establishment of a group practice in Albuquerque. Despite the fame and success of the Mayo model, group practice was anathema to many American physicians of the twenties and thirties. Solo practice remained "the American way," and in an era nearly obsessed with the fear of socialism and communism, the idea of cooperative efforts in medicine was unsettling and threatening to many Americans. Many private practitioners were alarmed by the possible competitive advantages of group practice, and straightforward economic self-interest was undoubtedly a major element in the hostility many solo physicians displayed toward the group-practice innovators.

The connection between the founding of a group practice and the development of intense hostility toward Dr. Lovelace, in particular, was an unmistakable one. Until 1929, he was a pillar of the Albuquerque medical establishment, fully integrated within it. (Dr. Lassetter, as suggested in chapter 1, had a much more tenuous relationship with the medical establishment.) The records of the Bernalillo County Medical Association, which later became a bastion of the anti-Lovelace forces, testify to Dr. Lovelace's initial full acceptance by the organization. For example, he was president of the medical association in 1916, read papers on a regular basis at its meetings,[17] held the group's monthly meetings in his home, and served frequently on its committees. But the Lovelace-Lassetter team's determination to establish a group practice drove a wedge between them and many other Albuquerque doctors, and the

17. "Ectopic Gestation" (5 May 1915); "Renal Calculi" (14 February 1923) and "The Surgical Aspects of Cavity Sterilization in Pulmonary Tuberculosis" (7 November 1923), among other papers, represented his contribution to the group's scientific discussions. See Bernalillo County Medical Association, Minutes for the dates cited.

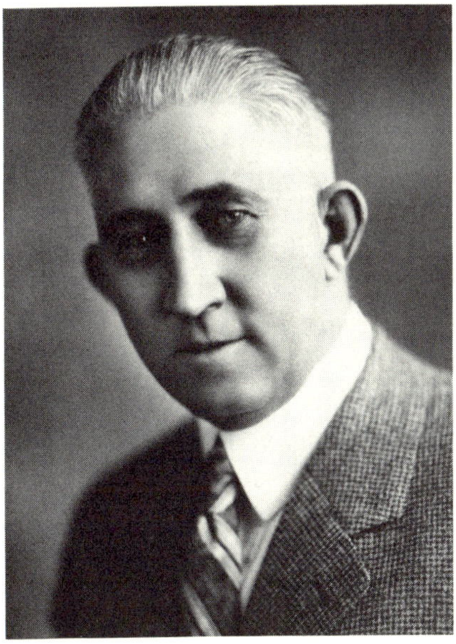

Dr. Lassetter in the late 1930s.

downtown docs were quick to express their displeasure. The excitement over "advertising" was quickly followed by another difficulty, which arose when Dr. Lamon sought membership in the local medical society. Applications such as his—where all the credentials were indisputably in order—were always approved pro forma and, except in extremely rare cases, by unanimous vote. Dr. Lamon was accepted for membership in the group, but only by a narrow tally of sixteen for, and eight against his admission. The vote was intended not so much as an insult toward Dr. Lamon personally, as it was directed toward his employers and what his presence in town represented.[18]

Despite this show of displeasure by their peers within the Albuquerque medical community, Drs. Lovelace and Lassetter

18. Dr. Lamon stayed with the Lovelace Clinic for thirteen years, until going off to war in 1942. He did not return thereafter, possibly because "he didn't get along with Randy and resented his taking over the place" (private communication with the author). For the remainder of his career he was in private practice in San Jose, California, dying there in 1979.

pushed ahead with their group-practice plans. Later in 1929, they hired a pediatrician, Jacob Travis Bennett, and a radiologist, Erwin Johns, to join their team. Like Lamon, both Bennett and Johns were highly skilled specialists with impeccable credentials in their fields. Bennett had earned his medical degree in 1926 at Baltimore's Johns Hopkins, possibly America's most distinguished medical school of the 1920s; then, he had trained in pediatrics at several of the most recognized children's hospitals on the East Coast. Similarly, Dr. Johns, a 1923 graduate of the University of Minnesota Medical School, had trained in his radiology specialty at the Mayo Clinic, and had done other postgraduate work on the continent; his acquisition by the Lovelace Clinic was a coup for the small, obscure group.[19] Both Bennett and Johns were among the founding members when their respective specialty boards were established in 1933 and 1934. Their hiring initiated a particular pattern of expansion that prevailed throughout the 1930s: when the clinic added a doctor, it selected only specialists representing the major subdisciplines of medicine and, when possible, it hired only graduates from medical institutions which supposedly guaranteed the best that American medicine had to offer. (However, even when pursuing the best physicians available, Dr. Lovelace's tough-fisted business principles lurked just below the surface—as the following telegram displays.)

Lee Monroe Miles, an obstetrician and gynecologist with outstanding credentials—he had already published extensively in his field, done graduate training at Johns Hopkins, and served on the teaching faculty at the Marquette University School of Medicine—was added to the staff in 1931;[20] and Stuart Adler, a pediatrician educated at Harvard and trained in some of the finest East Coast medical institutions as well as the Mayo Clinic,

19. Dr. Bennett stayed with the clinic for three years, and then departed for El Paso, where he was in private practice for the next half-century. Before his early death in 1940, Erwin Johns established a brilliant reputation as one of the pioneers of radiology in New Mexico.

20. Prior to his death in 1956, Dr. Miles devoted a full quarter-century of his life to the clinic. He was one of the fixtures of the place, beloved by his patients and respected by his colleagues. He served twenty-five years as head of the clinic's Obstetrics-Gynecology Department, and his portrait hangs in that department today.

Form 3385-B

THE WESTERN UNION TELEGRAPH COMPANY

TELEGRAM RECEIVED BY TELEPHONE

CHECK — OFFICE FROM — DATE — FILING TIME

ALBUQUERQUE, N. MEX.
APRIL 2, 1930.

DR. W. B. FIROR.
CARE OF DEPARTMENT OF ROENTGENOLOGY,
UNIVERSITY OF MICHIGAN.
ANN ARBOR, MICHIGAN.

WE ARE JUST STARTING OUR CLINIC THERE WILL BE VERY LITTLE WORK FOR SOME TIME FOR THAT REASON WE COULD NOT PAY MORE THAN THREE HUNDRED PER MONTH FOR FIRST YEAR THREE FIFTY PER MONTH FOR THE SECOND YEAR FOUR HUNDRED PER MONTH FOR THIRD YEAR AFTER THAT AN INCREASE IF EVERYTHING IS SATISFACTORY DEPENDING UPON THE AMOUNT OF WORK WE ARE DOING STOP HAVE A NEW SNOOK JUST INSTALLED WE WOULD WANT YOU AT ONCE IF POSSIBLE KINDLY WIRE IF INTERESTED REFERENCE FIRST NATIONAL BANK.

DR. W. R. LOVELACE.

CHG SIG.

SIGN — TELEPHONE NUMBER — CLASS OF STATION — SPECIAL INFORMATION

SENDER'S NAME

A 1930 telegram, carefully preserved at the Lovelace Clinic, illustrating the strong business sense of the senior Dr. Lovelace. (Dr. Firor refused the offer.)

joined the group in 1933.[21] William H. Thearle, a thoracic surgeon and a member of the founders' group of the American Board of Surgery, was affiliated with the clinic in 1934. Later in the decade came board-certified or eligible specialists in ear, nose and throat, internal medicine, and urology; several of them were the first such specialists in their fields to establish practices in New Mexico. The clinic remained numerically small—it grew from the two founders in 1929 to five members in 1931, eight in 1934, and ten in 1939—but nonetheless, its progress was noteworthy. Its staff in 1939 included three board-certified

21. Dr. Adler spent seven years at the Lovelace Clinic before a stint in the New Mexico Department of Health, and then devoted a quarter-century to private practice in Albuquerque. He was one of the most influential figures of organized medicine in New Mexico, serving as president of the state medical society in 1956–57 and as one of the organization's senior statesmen for years thereafter.

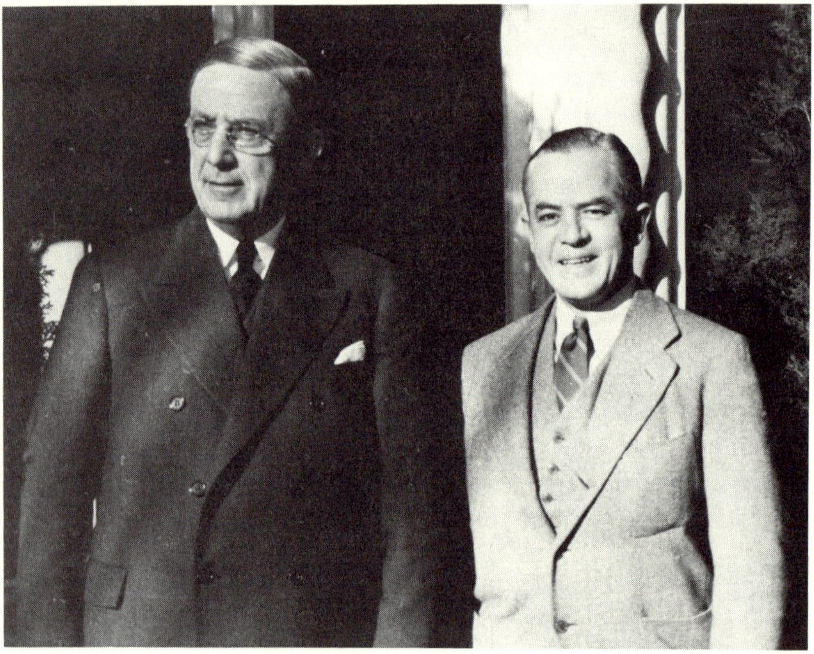

Dr. Lovelace and Dr. Charles W. Mayo in 1939 on one of the latter's frequent visits to Albuquerque.

surgeons (Drs. Lovelace, Lamon, and Thearle); board-certified specialists in obstetrics and gynecology, radiology, pediatrics, internal medicine, and ear, nose, and throat (Drs. Miles, Johns, Adler, H. Linton January, and T. H. Gallivan, respectively), as well as Dr. Lassetter. Within the broad spectrum of the development of medicine in New Mexico (and the Southwest generally), the Lovelace Clinic was one of the central agents in bring specialty medicine to the region. When the first *Directory of Medical Specialists* was published in 1939, six of the sixteen men listed in New Mexico practiced at the Lovelace Clinic, and two additional board-certified doctors joined the clinic's staff before the end of that year.

Associated with the addition of specialty-care staff or capability at the clinic was the development of its regional reputation as a referral center. Throughout the thirties, the Lovelace Clinic remained, of course, essentially a general-care institution serving the growing market of Albuquerque and its environs;

but as its specialist staff increased, it extended its influence to encompass most of the state of New Mexico and significant portions of adjacent states. Country doctors around the region were increasingly conscious of the Albuquerque institution as a place of high-quality specialty assistance; and, as highways were built and other communications improved, the Lovelace Clinic attracted rising numbers of patients referred from around the region. It was a development particularly welcomed and encouraged by Dr. Lovelace. He was well known for the assiduousness with which he "worked the countryside." He cultivated the friendship of the region's country-doctor populace, making sure that they were fully aware of the special services and support which his group could provide for them and their patients.[22] His leadership role in bringing specialty medicine to the state proved to be a two-edged sword, of course. It undoubtedly helped to raise the caliber of practice in, first, Albuquerque, and then, in the state, but it also increased the hostility toward the clinic from some physicians in and around Albuquerque. By bringing in board-certified specialists, the Lovelace Clinic was implicitly raising the question of the competency and caliber of practice among other physicians in the community, at least in particular cases. The development introduced questions about proper range of practice and even about ethics which had not previously concerned Albuquerque doctors.

This first phase of the history of the Lovelace Clinic—the time of its birth and early elaboration—reached its climax in 1941 with the hiring of six new men to fill out the group's staff. For several reasons, it was a special moment in the clinic's history. Physically, the additional staff made it necessary to rent the entire third floor of the downtown bank building and to begin initial planning for expansion into adjacent property. The increase in the professional staff to fourteen members,

22. This was the consistent testimony of the many New Mexico physicians I interviewed as part of the New Mexico Medical History Program, including more than two dozen practitioners who established their New Mexico careers in the 1930s. For example, Dr. Demarious Badger, of Hobbs, remembered that at medical meetings the two people who unfailingly made a point of greeting and chatting with her were the Drs. Lovelace, Uncle Doc and his nephew Randy. Dr. Demarious Badger, interview with the author, Albuquerque, 2 September 1983.

made the Albuquerque institution the largest single concentration of medical manpower in the entire Southwest, and extended its specialty coverage to include eight different fields. This 1941 expansion also underscored the clinic's commitment to bringing the best possible doctors to the region. All six of the new staff members were specialty-trained physicians whose credentials rivaled those of new recruits at the country's finest medical centers. For example, two of the new men came from the Mayo Clinic; another was from Harvard's Peter Bent Brigham Hospital training program; and a fourth had completed advanced studies at Chicago's Research and Education and Michael Reese hospitals.

Just as important, the Lovelace "class of 1941" brought stability to the staff. In the first decade of the clinic's existence, a number of staff physicians came and went in the downtown bank building. To be sure, some physicians remained with the Lovelace-Lassetter nucleus: Drs. Lamon (for thirteen years), Adler (seven years), Miles (twenty-five years), Johns (eleven years, until his death), Thearle (twenty-three years), and January (eighteen years). But others stayed for only brief periods of time at the Albuquerque clinic. During that first decade, nine other doctors arrived, stayed a while, and left, averaging only a year and a half with the clinic. Such a turnover was not particularly unusual when compared to the experience of group practices elsewhere in the country,[23] but nonetheless, it was a cause for concern. Some doctors (and their families) did not adapt well to the still semiexotic social, cultural, and physical environment of the isolated desert town. Others grew dissatisfied with the loss of independence inherent in a group practice, and almost everyone was unhappy with the pay scales of the Lovelace Clinic. Until his final days, Dr. Lovelace I was notoriously penurious with his money and remained reluctant to concede the necessity of paying his professional staff top

23. See Fred W. Wasserman and Michael C. Miller, *Building A Group Practice* (Springfield, Ill.: Charles C. Thomas, 1973), pp. 27–30 and Center For Research in Ambulatory Health Care Adminstration, *The Organization and Development of a Medical Group Practice* (Cambridge, Mass.: Ballinger Publishing Co., 1976), chapter 1.

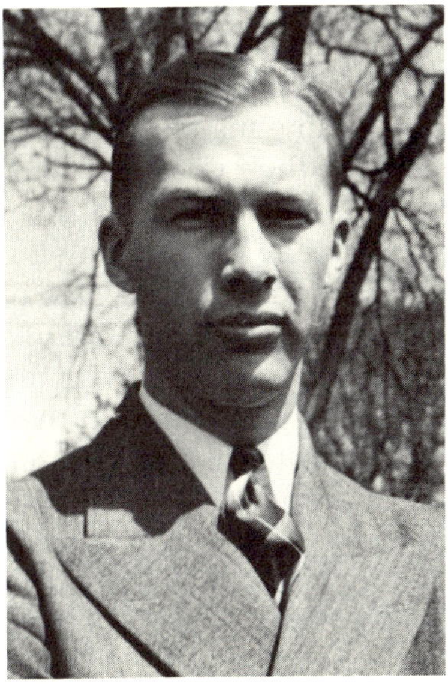

Dr. D. Angus McKinnon, general surgeon at the Lovelace Clinic, 1941–1976.

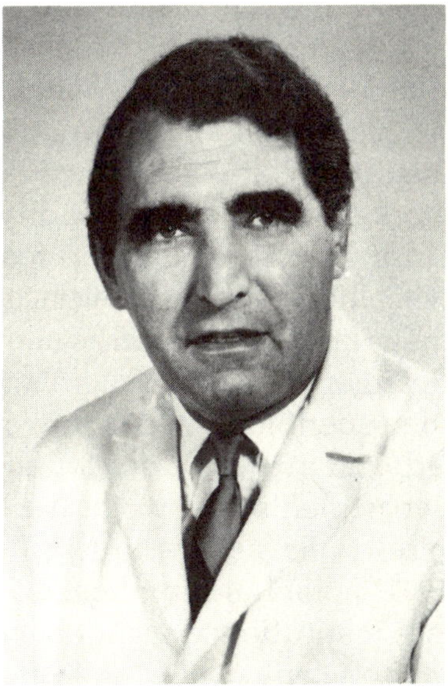

Dr. Jack Grossman, chief of radiology at the Lovelace Clinic, 1941–1971.

wages.[24] Unsurprisingly, as long as his influence was strong at the clinic, his attitude played a major part in a staff turnover of considerable scale.

But the group that arrived in 1941 was different. Although their personal and professional backgrounds ranged across a wide spectrum, four of the six new doctors hired that year found a strong match between their own personal needs, interests, and preferences and the opportunities available within the Albuquerque institution. Each of them served thirty years or longer on the clinic's staff and established positions of high honor and respect both within the clinic itself and the New

24. Dr. Donald Kilgore, who first came to the clinic in 1953 when Uncle Doc was still an influential figure in its councils, remembers a number of occasions when the older man disdainfully exclaimed, "You can always hire more doctors!" Dr. Donald E. Kilgore, interview with the author, Albuquerque, 18 November 1985.

Mexico medical community at large. Drs. Ollie Cramer in (originally) general internal medicine and later gastroenterology, Charles Fishback in pediatrics, Jack Grossman in radiology, and Angus McKinnon in surgery quickly became mainstays of the institution, and to a considerable degree, their energies, hard work, and all-around solidity built the modern Lovelace Clinic. During the three decades following 1941, they were among the wheelhorses of the Lovelace center. For example, they gave of their time and counsel as members of the Lovelace Foundation's Board of Trustees; as members of the clinic's Board of Governors they spent long hours in worrying over its business; and they led, and in some cases founded, their own clinical and research departments—all while they served full schedules as patient-care clinicians. In direct and measurable ways this "class of 1941" notably strengthened the still young and vulnerable Lovelace institution. Psychologically, the simultaneous arrival of so many talented new staffers signaled that the new institution had come to stay and intended to pursue its goal of excellence in medical care more vigorously than ever.

THREE

The Vision of Randy Lovelace

THE WAR YEARS INTERRUPTED the steady and unique growth of the Lovelace Clinic, restricting further expansion and experimentation with its staff and structure. Several of the younger staff members were called into military service; and other physicians filled in—most of them on an explicitly temporary basis—to help in caring for the increasingly doctor-poor civilian populace. Between 1942 and 1945, ten different physicians spent brief tenures at the clinic, assisting the nucleus of six to eight regular staff members who bore most of the patient load.[1] The momentum created by the clinic's steady expansion in the thirties gradually dissipated, and as the war wore on the institution's future grew increasingly uncertain.

The new men hired in 1941 and the older doctors who had joined the staff in the thirties could be relied upon to carry the institution forward after the war ended; but the clinic's adjustment to the postwar world require continued strong leadership. Dr. Lassetter was seventy-one years old and in declining health as the war drew to a close, and he could not be expected to play a major role in reshaping the clinic's future. (He died not long afterward, in 1948.) Dr. Lovelace, who was already accustomed to the leader's role in the partnership, was a robust

1. Dr. Robert C. Derbyshire, another board-certified surgeon who came early to New Mexico, practiced at the clinic from 1942 to 1948. A recovering tubercular, and thus exempt from military service, Dr. Derbyshire remembered the crushing patient loads of the period from 1943–1946, loads so heavy that he contemplated somehow escaping to military service for relief. Dr. Robert C. Derbyshire, interview with the author, Albuquerque, 9 October 1982.

sixty-two years old in 1945, and he still thrived on his work; but even he must have looked to the changing future with some anxiety.

The Second World War was a climacteric for American society, changing the norms of life in fundamental ways; and New Mexico was affected with special force by the changes that were set in motion. The federal government extended its presence in New Mexico with new or expanded military installations, laboratories, and the like; and large numbers of the state's young people were exposed to a war-torn world far beyond the perimeters of their native land. If nothing else, the war stripped New Mexico of its relative isolation and opened it to a much more intimate interchange with the humanity outside its borders. Dr. Lovelace was justifiably self-confident, but he must have known that a new vision would be indispensable as his clinic faced an uncertain future. That new vision came in the person of William Randolph Lovelace II. When the eleven-year-old Randy came to live with him during the First World War, the elder Dr. Lovelace had begun to hope that his nephew would eventually follow in his footsteps, building on the reputation and institution that he had fashioned. In later years, Randy Lovelace remembered driving to house calls with his busy uncle; and a tacit understanding grew between them that the boy would follow his bachelor uncle in pursuing a medical career.

Randy Lovelace was the driving force in the ambitious transformation of the Lovelace Clinic in 1947, and the new institution that he helped to shape was, to a large degree, the product of his particular interests, experience, and personality. From 1947 until his death in 1965, the younger Lovelace dominated the Albuquerque institution that his uncles had created, and he put his personal stamp on it in unmistakable fashion. Emerson once suggested, "An institution is often the extended shadow of one man," and it would be difficult to imagine any institution for which that judgment was more true than the Lovelace Foundation for Medical Education and Research. The Albuquerque health-care center became Randy Lovelace's personal vehicle, the expression of his special genius. It was his vision, industry, and talent which brought the clinic regional, and then national, recognition as a medical center of first importance. The range and dimensions of his accomplishments, which are supported by the strong testimony of those who knew him well, make it clear that he possessed a personality of rare power and brilliance.

Born in Missouri, Randy Lovelace came to New Mexico as a babe in arms. He was reared on the working cattle ranches owned by his father near Fort Sumner, Willard, and Gran Quivira, New Mexico, as well as in his Uncle Doc's house in Albuquerque. From his boyhood experiences on his father's ranch lands he developed a respect and affection for the rough, semidesert New Mexico countryside which was to mark his life. (When he was busiest, he liked to relax by hunting, fishing, or driving fast across the wide-open New Mexico landscape that he knew so well.)[2] In his uncle's home, in addition to a commitment to medicine, he was instilled with a desire to excel: to set high and worthy goals for his life and then to work ceaselessly toward their achievement. This ambition to do great things—or put it another way, the determination not to settle for the ordinary—was combined in Randy Lovelace with the willingness to dare to seek the extraordinary and to spend the effort necessary in achieving it. These attributes of character were the gifts of his uncle.

Little about his boyhood and adolescence was exceptional, but two aspects of his youth emphatically influenced the direction that his life took. First, the extended exposure to his strong-willed physician-uncle is an influence whose importance in shaping his future cannot be exaggerated. Second, a keen interest in things mechanical—how things worked and what made them work—extended far beyond the norms of little-boy or adolescent curiosity, and was most evident in his peculiarly strong fascination with flying. His personal friend and biographer, Richard G. Elliott, has speculated that Randy's fascination with flight and flying machines must have begun in his boyhood.[3] Documents show that he earned his wings as a twenty-

2. C. R. Smith, longtime president and guiding spirit of American Airlines and a close personal friend of Randy, remembered taking high-speed, curve-challenging auto trips with Randy at the wheel and the joy in the release that it afforded him. C. R. Smith, interview with the author, Washington, D.C., 7 January 1985.

3. Richard G. Elliott, " 'On a Comet, Always,' A Biography of Dr. William Randolph Lovelace II," *New Mexico Quarterly* 36, no. 4(1966–67):355–56.

year-old Navy ROTC cadet at Great Lakes Naval Training Center in the spring of 1928. Later that year, he wanted to accept the Navy's invitation to undergo advanced flight training at the Pensacola, Florida, Naval Air Station, but his Uncle Doc said no, insisting that it would be an unwarranted disruption of his education. However, his interest in aviation remained a constant part of his life. In his senior year in college, he coauthored a play, "Gold Feathers," which has been described as a story of aviation life "as told by a licensed pilot."[4]

After graduation in 1925 from Albuquerque High School—where his classmates voted him *least* likely to succeed—he attended Washington University in St. Louis, where he took his baccalaureate in 1930 with grades that were acceptable, though not brilliant. From premedical studies he moved on to medical school at the same institution; then, briefly, Cornell University Medical School; and finally, Harvard. Exposure to the remarkable men of the Harvard staff cemented his dedication to medicine and perhaps first stirred his interest in medical research. When he graduated in 1934 from Harvard, he left immediately for New York City and an internship at Bellevue Hospital. While in New York, he determined to focus on surgery, intending initially to seek a surgical residency at Bellevue. His uncle, however, had other ideas and urged him to consider advanced study at the Mayo Clinic; and a quick visit to the Rochester institution convinced Randy that the elder Dr. Lovelace was right in his boundless respect for the place. At the end of 1935, he was offered a fellowship in surgery at the Mayo Clinic, and in the following summer, he moved to Rochester. During the formative years of his surgical and medical-research career, his destiny was linked to that of one of America's most famous medical institutions.

Randy Lovelace's tenure at the Mayo Clinic was remarkably successful and, in some respects, spectacular. In pursuing his surgical specialization, he earned his M.S. degree in surgery from the Mayo Foundation of the University of Minnesota in 1939. In the process, he became an adept general surgeon with

4. Ibid., pp. 357–59.

a particular interest in thyroid and neck surgery.[5] As a practicing surgeon he possessed first-rate skills, but he never focused his abilities and energies entirely on surgery and thus never challenged the preeminent luminaries in the field. He is not remembered for any special technical artistry, nor for any imaginative or innovative contributions to his discipline. However, he passed the Mayo test with flying colors, winning the Mayo Foundation's coveted J. William White Scholarship in 1939, a grant awarded to particularly promising young surgeons to allow them to travel and study in major European surgical centers. In 1939–40, he was appointed as first assistant to Dr. Charles W. Mayo; and he was designated as a Mayo surgical chief in 1941.[6] From the late thirties and into the sixties he established a well-earned reputation as a competent, effective surgeon. But the surgical theater was not the arena where Randy Lovelace made his most indelible mark.

Far more important than his surgical work and training at the Mayo Clinic was the opportunity he found there to fuse his interests in aviation and medicine. At Mayo Randy had the chance to develop the interest in medical research, particularly in the field of aviation medicine, first kindled in him by his teachers at Harvard. At Mayo, he came under the influence of Dr. Walter M. Boothby, one of the authentic pioneers of aviation medicine. Dr. Boothby, whose work on metabolism and respiration made him one of the giants of the field, had begun his experimental work in Boston at Peter Bent Brigham Hospital and Harvard Medical School. In 1916, however, he moved to the Mayo Foundation, where he spent the next thirty-two years of his life. He was at the peak of his scientific activity and stature when Randy Lovelace first met him in 1937; and he was in the initial stages of organizing the famous Mayo Aero Medical Unit,

5. He had plans to write a general textbook on neck surgery, and the photographic files of the Lovelace Medical Foundation contain several thousand clinical photographs that he collected for that purpose over nearly a quarter-century.

6. Dr. Charles W. "Chuck" Mayo, son of founder Dr. Will Mayo, became a close friend of Randy, often visiting him (and his uncle) in Albuquerque and spending much time with him elsewhere as their medical careers crossed. His affection and high regard for Randy Lovelace are portrayed in his autobiography, *Mayo: The Story of My Family and My Career* (Garden City N.Y.: Doubleday and Co., 1968).

a research group that made fundamental contributions to American medical research during the Second World War.[7] The close and fruitful collaboration between the young surgeon and the experienced researcher was stimulated by two events earlier in 1937 that brought Randy Lovelace into closer contact with the world of aviation. In the first months of 1937 he applied for training as a flight surgeon, and after a course of study at Randolph Field, Texas, achieved that objective as well as the rank of first lieutenant in the U.S. Army Medical Corps Reserves. Later in the year, at the National Air Races in Cleveland, he met the extraordinary Jacqueline Cochran, already a world-renowned aviatrix, and a lifelong friendship ensued.[8]

The flight surgeon's training and his exposure through Jackie Cochran to the world of aviation daredevilry, when combined with the opportunity to work at Mayo with one of the luminaries of aviation medicine, transfixed the young surgeon from New Mexico, sealing an interest in aviation and then aerospace medicine which would endure for the rest of his life. Dr. Boothby immediately put him to work as a part of the Mayo Aero Medical Unit, which was then focused upon a study of the problems encountered by military and civilian pilots in flying in higher altitudes. Anoxia—or, more accurately, hypoxia—was one of the more acute and life-threatening dangers encountered by these pilots, and the Mayo researchers started to work on the task of devising an oxygen mask suitable for high-altitude flight. In relatively short order, the Mayo team—composed centrally of Drs. Boothby and Lovelace, and a third Mayo scientist and medical educator, Dr. Arthur Bulbulian—invented a unique oxygen mask, which Randy Lovelace personally tested in flights up to fifteen thousand feet in a single-engine Stinson piloted

7. Dr. Boothby retired from the Mayo Clinic in 1948, moving to Albuquerque not long afterward. He hoped that the arid climate would ease his asthma, and his former pupil and colleague, Dr. Lovelace II, wanted his help in getting underway the research operations of the new Lovelace Medical Foundation. Dr. and Mrs. Boothby lived in a guest house, adjacent to Randy Lovelace's home, which was specially constructed for them. He died on 4 July 1953.

8. Miss Cochran's husband, financier Floyd Odlum, also became Randy's close personal friend in the late 1930s, and a decade later he accepted Randy's request that he serve as the first president of the Lovelace Foundation's Board of Trustees.

by an industrialist friend, Henry H. Timken, Jr., of Dayton. (Years later, Timken became a trustee of the Lovelace Medical Foundation.)[9]

The first public announcement of the new mask—called the BLB mask after its inventors Boothby, Lovelace, and Bulbulian—came at the tenth annual meeting of the Aero Medical Association, held in Dayton, Ohio, in September 1938. The report presented by the Mayo researchers, entitled "Oxygen in Aviation: The Necessity for the Use of Oxygen and a Practical Apparatus for Its Administration to Both Pilots and Passengers," immediately attracted wide attention. The BLB mask, which was the central focus of the report, quickly became the first generally accepted oxygen-breathing apparatus for high-altitude flight, and for years it was standard equipment in both military and commercial aircraft.[10] Randy Lovelace's role in the mask's development, together with his contributions to other research at the Mayo Aero Medical Unit on pilot fatigue, nitrogen elimination, and the air transport of patients with pneumothorax, established his name prominently in the developing field of aviation medical research. One tangible sign of the thirty-two-year-old Mayo surgeon's "arrival" was his recognition as one of the 1940 recipients of the Robert J. Collier Trophy, an award given each year "for the greatest achievement in aviation in America, the value of which has been thoroughly demonstrated by actual use during the preceding year." In December 1940, President Franklin Delano Roosevelt presented this prized aeronautical honor to the airlines of the United States for their high record of safety, with special recognition to Drs. Boothby and Lovelace and U.S. Army Captain Harry G. Armstrong for

9. One of Randy Lovelace's more striking characteristics was the way in which he bound friends to himself, including many with whom he had only relatively casual associations. Earl D. Johnson (former president of General Dynamics and aviation consultant), interview with the author, Greenwich, Conn., 6 January 1985.

10. For good, detailed accounts of the development of the BLB mask within the context of aviation medical research, see Eloise Engle and Arnold S. Lott, *Man in Flight: Biomedical Achievements in Aerospace* (Annapolis, Md.: Leeward Publications, Inc., 1979), pp. 64–66 and Ross A. McFarland, *Human Factors in Air Transportation: Occupational Health and Safety* (New York: McGraw-Hill Book Co., Inc., 1953), pp. x–xi. For these references I am grateful to Dr. Clayton S. White.

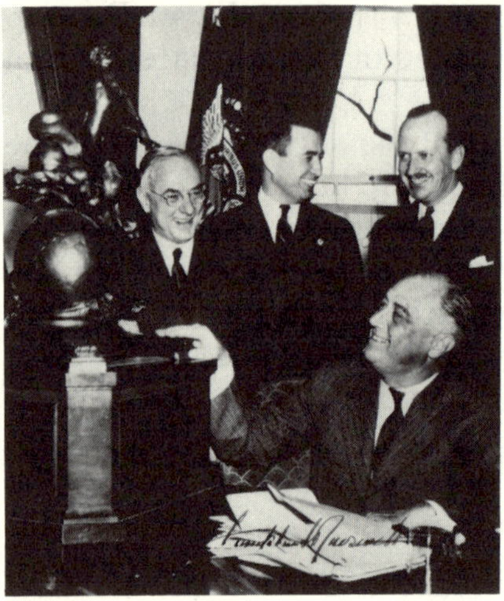

Presentation of the Robert J. Collier Trophy by President Franklin Roosevelt in 1940. Standing in the center, behind the president, is Randy Lovelace, with Dr. Boothby to his right and U.S. Army Captain Harry G. Armstrong to his left.

their individual contributions to aviation medicine, in general, and to the problem of pilot fatigue, in particular.

After the landmark work on the BLB mask and a tour of European surgical centers that followed, Dr. Lovelace settled into his surgical work at Mayo, and continued his explorations in aviation medicine. With America's entry into the Second World War, he was redirected to focus exclusively on his research. In February 1942, Major Lovelace was assigned as assistant director of research in the Office of the Air Surgeon in Washington, D.C. Three months later, he managed to arrange reassignment to a research position at the Aero Medical Laboratory at Wright Field, Ohio, as a kind of troubleshooter traveling to the war's operational theaters to check on the functionality of various items of aeromedical personal equipment in wartime use. He then served briefly as chief of the laboratory's Oxygen Branch, and finally as chief of the Aero Medical Laboratory from July 1943 until his release from the service in March 1946.

During this highly productive period at the Aero Medical Laboratory, Colonel Lovelace performed a piece of old-fashioned derring-do that won for him the Distinguished Flying Cross. As the war progressed, the special problems of military pilots facing the necessity of bailout at high altitudes received increasing attention. The dangers inherent in that endeavor—most obviously oxygen deprivation in the upper layers of the atmosphere—urgently demanded the attention of aeromedical researchers. Colonel Lovelace and his team at Wright Field soon designed prototype equipment that they thought would handle the problem. However, their experimental gear, basically a small bailout cylinder containing an approximately twelve-minute supply of oxygen, clearly needed to be tested in the field. Though Randy Lovelace had extensive experience in flying, he had never taken a parachute jump in his life. Nevertheless, he decided to take the crucial first high-altitude leap himself, rather than assign the dubious honor to one of his subordinates.[11] Less than three months earlier, soon after his appointment as chief of the laboratory, he had received a letter from his Uncle Doc in Albuquerque, which had closed with the following admonition:

> Now, son, what you must do is to guard against any unnecessary chances in getting injured. Your reputation is made and all you have to do is protect your health and the rest will be o.k.[12]

This time Randy Lovelace felt compelled to ignore his uncle's advice. On 24 June 1943, he made his historic parachute leap, a jump which received extensive national press coverage, including pictures and articles in *Life* and *Look* magazines, among other places. To demonstrate the dependability of the portable oxygen system developed by his laboratory, he dropped through the bomb bay of a B-17 laboring to hold 40,200 feet of altitude

11. The air force experimenters projected a jump from forty-thousand feet as an appropriate test for the new equipment. Only once previously in history had any man successfully attempted bailout from such a height. A Russian army major reportedly had jumped from 40,813 feet, but had free fallen to 2,100 feet before opening his chute—and he had done this on his 599th jump. It was planned that Colonel Lovelace would open his chute immediately to avoid the risk of blackout associated with hypoxia—and because this would be his first experience with parachuting. Shirley Thomas, *Men of Space: Profiles of the Leaders in Space Research, Development, and Exploration* (Philadelphia and New York: Chilton Company, 1960–65), vol. 2, pp. 89–90.

12. William Randolph Lovelace I, Albuquerque, to WRL II, Wright Field, Ohio, 2 April 1943, in WRL I historical file, Lovelace Medical Foundation archives.

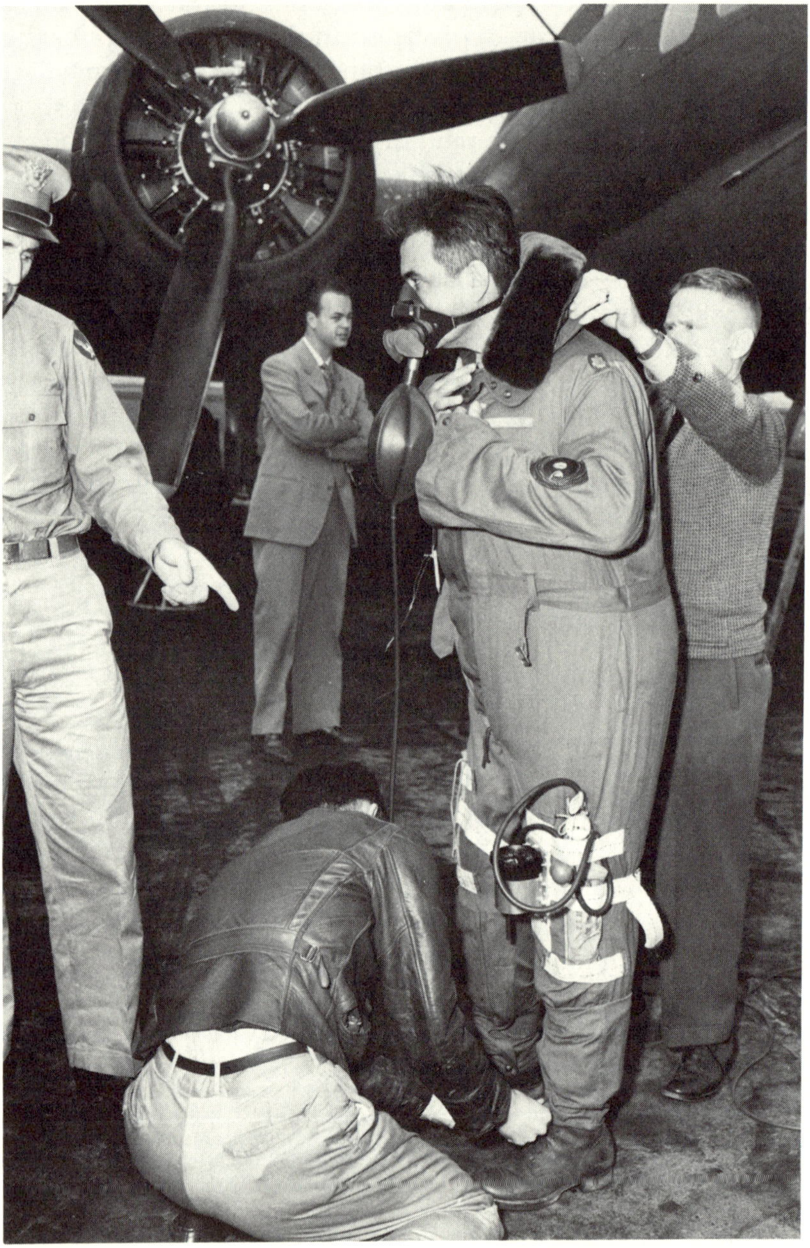

Colonel Randy Lovelace preparing for his experimental parachute jump, 24 June 1943.

above the wheatfields of central Washington State. Garbed in a suit specially rigged by team members in Ohio, he wore a back-type parachute, which was attached to a static line in the aircraft, as well as a chest-type, fail-safe parachute. The official War Department report, in an improvement upon its usual prose, described the jump:

> Colonel Lovelace climbed down onto a seat in the bomb bay to face the rear, leaned forward, and turned on the bail-out oxygen supply. Miles away he saw the Columbia River, a thin, shining ribbon twisting through fields of green. Thirty thousand feet below, a liaison plane moved along its course, ready to follow the jumper to earth. As his plane sped forward at 200 miles per hour, Colonel Lovelace stepped off into air 50° below zero. The tail of the plane was directly over his head when the chute started to open. The blast of onrushing air and the sudden jerk of the opening parachute tore the thick outer glove from both his hands and also snapped off the thin inner glove on his left hand, leaving it bare in freezing temperature. The inner glove remained on his right hand which was uninjured by the cold.[13]

The test protocol had been structured on the premise that there would be less shock if the chute were opened in thin, high air than if it were opened at a lower altitude. However, the opposite proved to be true. It was later estimated that Colonel Lovelace experienced a force of 30 to 40 Gs of pressure when the chute opened, with the jolt knocking him unconscious. As the chase plane watched in horror, he dangled like a pendulum bob, describing giant arcs through the air. After more than fifteen minutes of descent, during which he showed no signs of life, he roused at eight thousand feet, waved feebly to the chase plane, and finally landed hard in a field of wheat stubble. Too weak to handle the chute properly, he tumbled and was dragged along the ground. Several years later, a writer

13. Cited in Robert Joseph Benford, *Doctors in the Sky: The Story of the Aero Medical Association* (Springfield, Ill.: Charles Thomas Publishers, 1955), pp. 154–56.

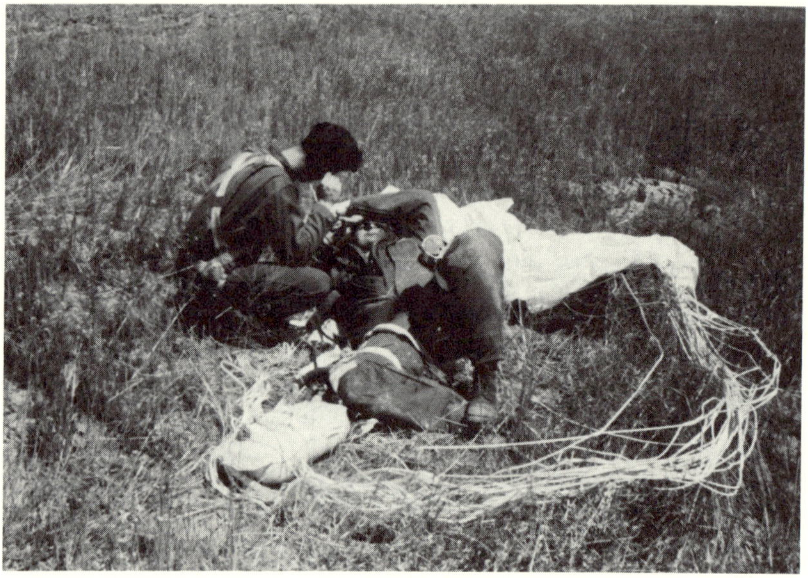

Immediately after the jump, a corpsman tends the shaken Colonel Lovelace, who holds his frostbitten left hand to his head.

who had the chance to interview both Dr. Lovelace and several other members of the test team described the last few minutes of this adventure and its overall significance:

> On the borderline of fuzzy consciousness, his doctor's instincts guided him to hold his left hand up to the sun's warmth. The pain of severe frostbite was becoming acute in this gloveless hand that had been exposed to 50° below zero temperature during the first part of his drop. The reaction of shock was setting in, and he was nauseated from the long period of swinging to and fro which he had undergone while unconscious. But even so, with trained objectivity, Lovelace was noting his own recovery. He was able to form sentences, but about one word in every sentence was difficult to pronounce. This he attributed to anoxia—the portable oxygen bottle had kept him alive during the descent, but it had not been sufficient to prevent a degree of anoxia. These effects he considered to

> be minor ones, however. One vital factor flooded his thoughts as he lay still weak in that wheat field—he now knew that the oxygen bottle had worked—had brought him to earth alive!
>
> What he was then too dazed to realize was that an even more significant part of his bail-out was the opening shock he had received. This proved all previous thinking in error. . . . In thinner air, the parachute opening shock was far greater—four times greater at 40,000 feet than at sea level. Though the experience had been unexpectedly hazardous for Lovelace, his test occasioned the laying down of new rules pertaining to jumping: in the event of emergency bail-out at high altitudes, there should be a delayed opening of the chute until the lower and denser altitudes, preferably 10,000-15,000 feet, had been reached. Thus had Lovelace advanced aviation medicine a giant step toward the fringes of space.[14]

After his landmark parachute jump, Colonel Lovelace spent nearly three full years as chief of the Aero Medical Laboratory at Wright Field, Ohio. During that time, he consolidated and extended his reputation as one of the leading figures in the rapidly expanding field of aviation medicine. Those years were also a time in which he made institutional and personal contacts that later proved to be of cardinal importance in shaping his own personal destiny as well as the future of the Albuquerque institution, which eventually he would head. With his experience in the Mayo Clinic and his first studies in aviation medicine, he was already well integrated in the world of clinical medicine and, even more so, in medical research. Throughout his variegated career, he was comfortable in those orbits and moved familiarly through them. From 1943 to 1946, he acquired a sure grasp of the structure and workings of the nation's military establishment and became part of an extensive network of professional contacts and friends within it. Those who knew him and watched him operate as head of the Lovelace Medical Foundation were invariably impressed with the way in which

14. Thomas, *Men of Space*, p. 91.

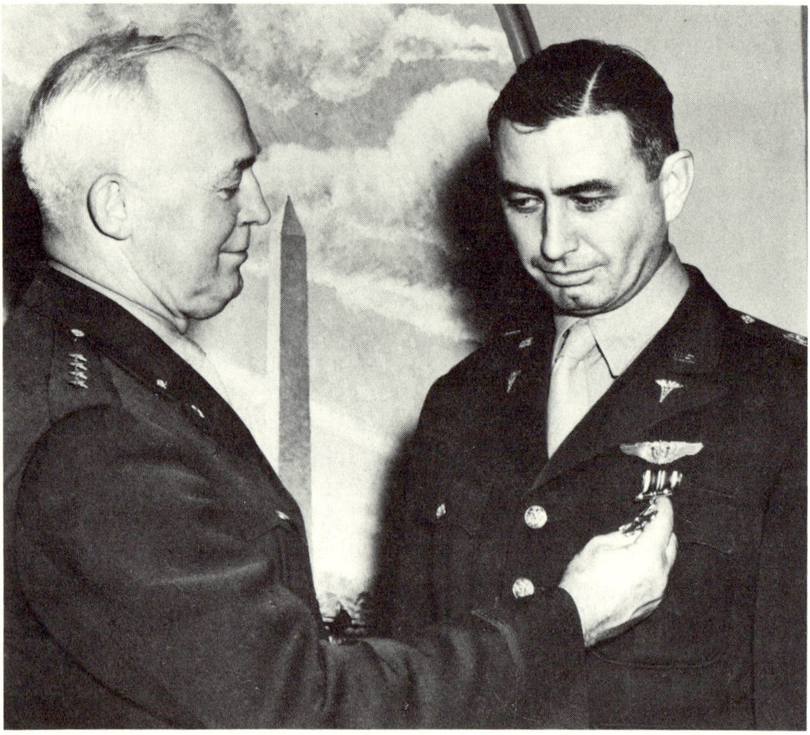

In late 1943, Colonel Lovelace received the Distinguished Flying Cross, presented here by General "Hap" Arnold (left).

he was able to move swiftly and easily through (and sometimes around) the government bureaucracy, relying on his knowledge of the system as well as the assistance of his personal acquaintances—all of which served the interests of the young and struggling foundation richly, especially during its early years.

In addition, he began to discover another group of allies during the war years, when the boundary lines between military and civilian aviation were hazy and sometimes nonexistent. Strategically located within the overall structure of things as head of the influential Aero Medical Laboratory, Dr. Lovelace made many friends who were already powerhouses in civilian aviation and in the aviation construction industry or who would become such in the postwar years. Floyd Odlum (whose service within the Lovelace institution will be discussed in detail later; see pp. 78–81) was one such person. A lawyer-financier of great power and influence when they first met at the Mayo Clinic, Odlum was a man who exerted a powerful influence on Dr. Lovelace. Married in 1936 to Jackie Cochran, Odlum became a major figure in America's aviation industry during the postwar era. He was the type of high-powered corporate tycoon and business executive, particularly within the aviation industry, that Randy Lovelace came to know well during the late thirties and the war years. Others included C. R. Smith, the founding father who built American Airlines to greatness; Earl Johnson, one-time president of General Dynamics as well as vice president of Delta Air Lines; and Thomas F. Ryan III, scion of an American family of legendary wealth and power and himself one of the financier-executives who put together and operated several different airline companies during the thirties, forties, and fifties. Men such as these became Randy Lovelace's friends during the late thirties and the Second World War; later he was able to enlist their help in supporting and directing the Lovelace Foundation for Medical Education and Research.

By the war's end, the young doctor from New Mexico had achieved extraordinary distinction and was close to the centers of power within several different spheres of American professional and corporate life. In the world of medicine, for example, he was a section chief at the Mayo Clinic and a researcher of world renown in the field of aviation medicine. He was also a well-connected figure in that important sector of American life that President Eisenhower would call, a few years later, the "military-industrial complex," especially in the areas of military and civilian aviation and construction. And he had made a marked success of his personal life as well. In the fall of 1933 he married Mary Easter Moulton, the lovely and accomplished daughter of a family prominent in New Mexico commercial circles. (Mary's father, Earl, like Uncle Doc Lovelace, was a victim of tuberculosis who had come to New Mexico for his health just after the turn of the century and had survived to become a major success as a businessman.) The union was a happy one, and Mary shared Randy's hectic, stimulating years

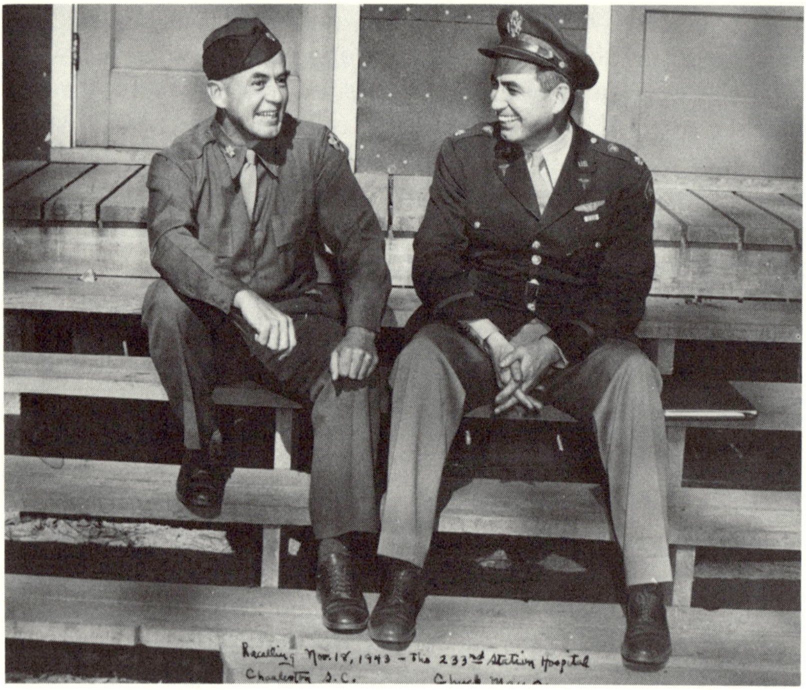
Recalling Nov. 18, 1943 – The 233rd Station Hospital
Charleston S.C.

Wartime photograph of Dr. Randy Lovelace with his friend Dr. Charles Mayo.

at Harvard, Bellevue, and Rochester, and then tolerated his extended absences during the war. Three children were born: Mary Christine, in 1938; William Randolph Lovelace III, in 1940; and Charles Moulton Lovelace in 1942.

When the surgeon-researcher, not yet forty, took terminal leave from the Army Air Corps in December 1945, his prospects seemed boundless. The obvious course of action was to return to the Mayo Clinic to resume the brilliant career that had been not so much interrupted as reoriented by the war. If he chose, he could return to the surgical practice which he had begun at Rochester almost a decade earlier. If research and research management were to become his main focus, supplemented perhaps by a limited surgical practice, the Mayo setup could also accommodate that kind of career. There is evidence, however, that he was under at least gentle pressure from his Uncle Doc in Albuquerque to consider returning home to assist in the job of reorienting the Lovelace Clinic and preparing it for the future.[15] Both Randy and Mary Lovelace were interested by that possibility, for both had a powerful sense of place as well as a special feeling of affection for their native state. For the short-term future, however, they decided to return to Rochester, while considering the various options open to them.

A personal tragedy of almost unbearable dimensions ultimately made up their minds for them. In early June of 1946, only a few months after the Lovelace family had resettled in Rochester, a polio epidemic then raging in the Minnesota citadel of modern medicine took the life of their five-and-a-half-year-old son. Despite the best efforts of Randy's colleagues on the Mayo staff, William Randolph Lovelace III died on 7 July. Randy telephoned his Uncle Doc, who was in San Francisco attending the annual convention of the American Medical Association, to tell him that the family intended to return the little boy to Albuquerque for burial. Within days of the burial service, four-year-old Chuckie Lovelace began to show unmistakable signs of the disease. Accompanied by his parents and sister, he was flown in Jackie Cochran's private plane from Albuquerque to Warm Springs, Georgia, for treatment at the foundation there; but in three weeks the second Lovelace son was dead. Stricken by this enormous tragedy, the bereaved family returned to Albuquerque. The Mayos wrote to Randy, urging him to return to Rochester to let work ease his grief, but he told Uncle Doc that he simply could not go back.[16] Through the remainder of that summer and early fall, he and Mary spent most of their time in the nearby Jémez mountains, with Randy occupying his time in fishing and chopping wood and Mary losing herself in the green peace of the mountains. Finally, Randy recommenced the tentative discussions begun earlier in the year with his Uncle Doc regarding the prospects for his return to Albuquerque and the Lovelace Clinic. The decision was soon reached: he and his family would return to Albuquerque, and with them a new era would begin for the Lovelace Clinic.

15. Elliott, " 'On a Comet, Always," ' p. 367; Dr. Clayton S. White, interview with the author, Albuquerque, 14 October 1985.

16. Elliott, " 'On a Comet, Always," ' p. 367.

Critical to Randy Lovelace's decision to return to Albuquerque was his uncle's agreement to a full-scale reorganization of the Lovelace Clinic. Specifically, on the base of the successful clinic he wanted to build a modern medical foundation committed to the triad of medical care, education, and research. The younger Dr. Lovelace was proud of the record that his uncles' clinic had established in providing top-quality health care, particularly in specialty medicine, to the people of Albuquerque and a broad swath of the Southwest. He did not wish to ignore or deemphasize that service in the future; and the record of the Lovelace Clinic during the eighteen years in which he was its director shows an enormous expansion of its staff and the services provided to its patients. He was an honest clinician and remained keenly aware that clinical medicine—the hands-on delivery of the best medical care possible—remained the essential foundation of the Lovelace Medical Center.[17]

But he wanted the Lovelace Clinic to do more than practice medicine, to be more than just another center of first-quality medical care. His experience at the Mayo Clinic had shown him what vision, energy, and boldness could make possible. He intended to fashion a medical center which fused the triad of patient care, education, and research in an integral way; and he was entirely convinced that New Mexico and the Southwest direly needed such an institution. Throughout the vast area stretching from Dallas-Fort Worth in the east to Los Angeles in the west, and from Denver to the Mexican border, there was not a single medical school; no hospitals or other institutions with approved internships; no residency programs of any sort for the training of physicians; only a handful of nursing schools

17. If, on occasion, that reality threatened to slip into the shadows of the educational and research programs in which Randy was so interested his Uncle Doc was always there to redress the balance. Thirty years after the fact, Dr. Robert U. Massey, a Lovelace staff member from 1951 to 1968, recalled: "Uncle Doc repeatedly reminded Randy that his base was the clinic, that he had to tend and build that base before he could go off to the moon—while Randy was already thinking, literally, about going to the moon." Dr. Robert U. Massey, interview with the author, Farmington, Conn., 4 January 1985. From Lovelace Clinic, Dr. Massey went on to become the dean of the University of Connecticut Medical School, where he served until his retirement in 1985.

turning out limited numbers of students (two schools in New Mexico produced eighty-five nursing graduates in 1947); and not a single approved program for the training of vital medical technical personnel such as X-ray technicians, dieticians, physical therapists, and medical technologists. In terms of medical education, the Southwest was a barren wasteland, entirely dependent on migration in acquiring trained medical personnel. There was clearly room, and indeed a critical need, for an institution that would help fill that void and serve as the medical educational hub for the entire region.

But there was more than an educational mission to be served by the expanded and redirected Lovelace medical center that Randy envisioned. He was also determined to push large-scale programs of medical research, particularly programs focused in his favorite field of aviation medicine. His commitment exceeded mere allegiance to the abstract idea that medical practice, education, and research ought to go forward together, with each area feeding and being fed by the others. He believed that, of course, but he also had more concrete reasons for his interest in an ambitious research program. With Dr. Boothby's impending retirement and departure from the Mayo Clinic and the predictable diminution in the importance of its Aero Medical Unit, Randy Lovelace was convinced that there was a need and an opportunity for a medical research institution with a special focus on aviation medicine. With his own strong reputation in the field and his extensive contacts throughout the defense establishment and the aviation industry, he felt that he might be able to capitalize on that opportunity. In Albuquerque, there were no laboratories, no support money, no staff, and few specific plans or proposals to support that kind of enterprise; but such constraints did not intimidate him. With the secure base of the Lovelace Clinic, he believed that much could be achieved: laboratory space could be scrounged or built; talented staff could be hired—and during his Mayo and military years, he had already identified a number of bright young researchers whom he might seek to lure to Albuquerque. In the flux of the immediate postwar years, many of them might be attainable; and with talented researchers would come the specific plans and imaginative proposals for new inquiries. In addition, the explosively changing world of aviation was producing almost daily new and lengthening lists of problems and challenges for the researchers in aviation medicine. Ideas and specific programs of work would pose no problem. He was confident (and time would prove him right) that he could enlist the support of his friends and colleagues in the aviation industry in the form of gifts and research contracts, as well as leads to other financial-support sources, and that their assistance would enable the institution to develop a powerful momentum. But those financial resources, though potentially great, would necessarily be secondary at the start. The base of the projected research, education, and patient-care center had to be the Lovelace Clinic.

There are no records of the discussions between young Dr. Lovelace and his two uncles regarding his dreams for the transformation of the Lovelace institution. Apparently, however, Randy experienced relatively little difficulty in persuading the older men to agree to the experiment that he had in mind. Dr. Lassetter, seventy-four years old and ill, had withdrawn, to a large degree, from active involvement in the clinic's affairs. His family was already well provided for, so he was prepared to make the personal financial sacrifice involved in converting the partnership into a foundation; and almost surely, he was relieved to know that the institution would go forward, albeit in radically changed form. Uncle Doc, too, was attracted by Randy's ideas. In 1947 he was sixty-four years old, and though far from longing for retirement, he was eager to share the load of leadership which he had borne so ably for a quarter-century. He had hoped that Randy would return to succeed him in directing the clinic; and the conditions the nephew imposed—the transformation of the place—were not at all alien to the older man's dreams. After all, it was Uncle Doc who had first come to esteem the Mayo operation and had steered his nephew toward it; so he could hardly have been surprised by, still less unsympathetic to, the dreams that Randy brought back with him to Albuquerque.

There was also an element of noblesse oblige, or genuine philanthropy, in the elder Lovelace's reaction. In a letter of acknowledgement sent to friends and well-wishers who wrote to congratulate him on the creation of the Lovelace Foundation, he responded: "I felt that it was only right that I should contribute something to the public from which it came in the past and will come in the future. The best in nature [New Mexico] and the best in medicine should go forward together, and we feel we have this."[18] To an old friend in Fort Sumner, a lawyer, he wrote, in a similar vein: "I feel that what I am trying to do will be beneficial to humanity in general, and, as I had regained my health in this state and I had accumulated a few dollars, it seemed only right to seek a way to return something."[19] But there was a distinctly different note sounded in another letter written at the same time, in which he acknowledged his taste for the challenge inherent in the new experiment:

> You can see now one of the reasons for the great tension I have been under for the past year, trying to put this deal over. . . . We have already been classified by my friends as the Mayo Clinic of the West. *I expect to continue directing this work as long as I am active. As you well know, this type of work has always been my first love.*[20]

Uncle Doc was far more practical and hardheaded than his gifted nephew, but even he was infected by Randy's enthusiasm and conviction that great things were possible. In addition, Randy had a proven track record. The dream that he shared with his Albuquerque uncles was ambitious indeed, but at Harvard, Bellevue, the Mayo Clinic, and the Aero Medical Laboratory he had set high goals for himself and then delivered. Uncle Doc was willing to let him take the lead, but he also intended to stay close to the center of things, prepared always to inject a note of caution or hard-nosed realism when he thought circumstances required it.

18. WRL I to John Murphy (manager of the Albuquerque Chamber of Commerce), 8 October 1947, in WRL I, Correspondence file, Lovelace Medical Foundation archives.

19. WRL I to Keith W. Edwards, Fort Sumner, 6 October 1947, in ibid.

20. WRL I to Mrs. Thomas L. Daily, Tucson, Ariz., 8 October 1947, in ibid. (Emphasis added.)

FOUR

Birth of the Lovelace Foundation

THROUGH THE FINAL MONTHS OF 1946 and the first half of 1947, preparations were made, particularly in arranging for the required legal work, to establish a new medical foundation on the base of the Lovelace Clinic. Because Rochester's Mayo organization was the explicit model for the institution taking shape in Albuquerque, the Mayo leadership and staff provided direct assistance to the Albuquerque planners, especially in defining the structural relationship between the Lovelace Clinic and the new Lovelace Foundation.[1] On several occasions, Dr. Lovelace II visited Rochester with his Albuquerque legal and business advisors (attorney D. A. MacPherson, Judge C. M. Botts, and accountant J. Bryan Stephenson) to work out details and to investigate the Mayo operation more closely.

The Mayo Clinic and Foundation was central to the establishment of the Lovelace Medical Foundation during the latter's formative years, serving as inspiration for the New Mexico institution; as the explicit model for its structure; and as its continuing ally and supporter. In recruiting new doctors, Lovelace usually called Mayo first. In determining, for example, the physical layout for a Department of Urology, the first step in resolving the problem was to send someone to Rochester to learn how they had done it there. In selecting the exact business form to use as a billing statement, the Mayo form was the first

1. Lovelace Medical Foundation, Board of Trustees, Minutes, 25 September 1947.

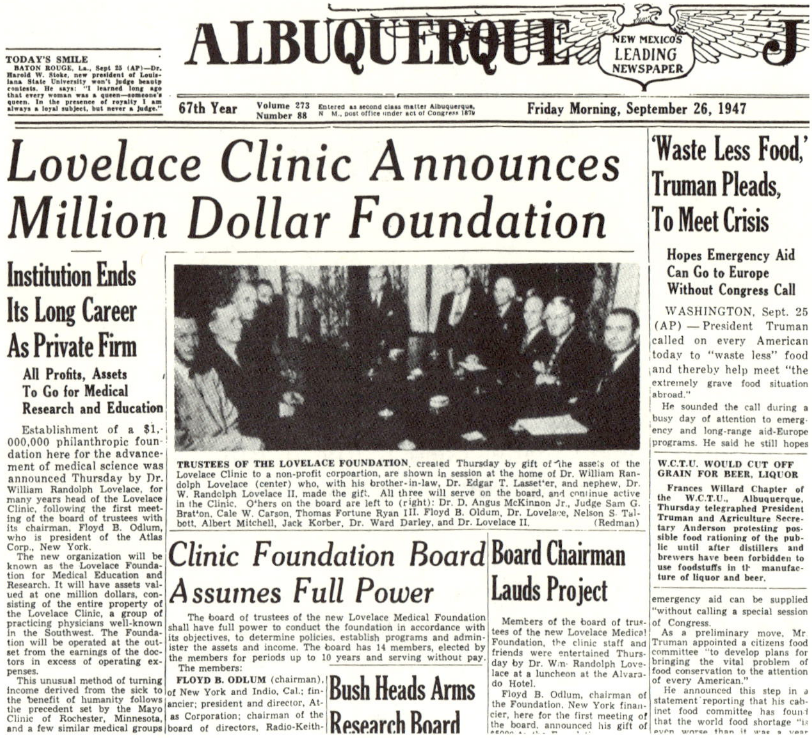

TODAY'S SMILE

BATON ROUGE, La., Sept 25 (AP)—Dr. Harold W. Stoke, new president of Louisiana State University won't judge beautp contests. He says: "I learned long ago that every woman was a queen—someone's queen. In the presence of royalty I am always a loyal subject, but never a judge."

ALBUQUERQUE J

NEW MEXICO'S LEADING NEWSPAPER

67th Year Volume 273 Number 88 Entered as second class matter Albuquerque, N. M., post office under act of Congress 1879 Friday Morning, September 26, 1947

Lovelace Clinic Announces Million Dollar Foundation

Institution Ends Its Long Career As Private Firm

All Profits, Assets To Go for Medical Research and Education

Establishment of a $1,-000,000 philanthropic foundation here for the advancement of medical science was announced Thursday by Dr. William Randolph Lovelace, for many years head of the Lovelace Clinic, following the first meeting of the board of trustees with its chairman, Floyd B. Odlum, who is president of the Atlas Corp., New York.

The new organization will be known as the Lovelace Foundation for Medical Education and Research. It will have assets valued at one million dollars, consisting of the entire property of the Lovelace Clinic, a group of practicing physicians well-known in the Southwest. The Foundation will be operated at the outset from the earnings of the doctors in excess of operating expenses.

This unusual method of turning income derived from the sick to the benefit of humanity follows the precedent set by the Mayo Clinic of Rochester, Minnesota, and a few similar medical groups

TRUSTEES OF THE LOVELACE FOUNDATION, created Thursday by gift of the assets of the Lovelace Clinic to a non-profit corpoartion, are shown in session at the home of Dr. William Randolph Lovelace (center) who, with his brother-in-law, Dr. Edgar T. Lasset'er, and nephew, Dr. W. Randolph Lovelace II, made the gift. All three will serve on the board, and continue active in the Clinic. O'hers on the board are left to (right): Dr. D. Angus McKinnon Jr., Judge Sam G. Brat'on, Cale W. Carson, Thomas Fortune Ryan III. Floyd B. Oldum, Dr. Lovelace, Nelson S. Talbott, Albert Mitchell, Jack Korber, Dr. Ward Darley, and Dr. Lovelace II. (Redman)

Clinic Foundation Board Assumes Full Power

The board of trustees of the new Lovelace Medical Foundation shall have full power to conduct the foundation in accordance with its objectives, to determine policies, establish programs and administer the assets and income. The board has 14 members, elected by the members for periods up to 10 years and serving without pay.

The members:

FLOYD B. ODLUM (chairman), of New York and Indio, Cal.; financier; president and director, Atlas Corporation; chairman of the board of directors, Radio-Keith-

Bush Heads Arms Research Board

Board Chairman Lauds Project

Members of the board of trustees of the new Lovelace Medical Foundation, the clinic staff and friends were entertained Thursday by Dr. Wm. Randolph Lovelace at a luncheon at the Alvarado Hotel.

Floyd B. Odlum, chairman of the Foundation, New York financier, here for the first meeting of the board, announced his gift of

'Waste Less Food,' Truman Pleads, To Meet Crisis

Hopes Emergency Aid Can Go to Europe Without Congress Call

WASHINGTON, Sept. 25 (AP) — President Truman called on every American today to "waste less" food and thereby help meet "the extremely grave food situation abroad."

He sounded the call during a busy day of attention to emergency and long-range aid-Europe programs. He said he still hopes emergency aid can be supplied "without calling a special session of Congress.

As a preliminary move, Mr. Truman appointed a citizens food committee "to develop plans for bringing the vital problem of food conservation to the attention of every American."

He announced this step in a statement reporting that his cabinet food committee has found that the world food shortage "is

W.C.T.U. WOULD CUT OFF GRAIN FOR BEER, LIQUOR

Frances Willard Chapter of the W.C.T.U., Albuquerque, Thursday telegraphed President Truman and Agriculture Secretary Anderson protesting possible food rationing of the public until after distillers and brewers have been forbidden to use foodstuffs in th manufacture of liquor and beer.

Front page of the *Albuquerque Journal*, 26 September 1947.

to be checked.[2] With Randy Lovelace's death in 1965, the ties between the two institutions began to wane, for to a considerable degree they were purely personal. In time, some Lovelace staffers came to dislike and even resent the relationship with Rochester that had once been so prominent. Nevertheless, in its early years at least, the Lovelace medical complex in Albuquerque bore the Mayo stamp in an emphatic way.

The lengthy discussion among the three partners of the Lovelace Clinic[3] and the careful legal work required in setting

2. See, for example, the Minutes of the Board of Governors, Lovelace Clinic, for 8 July 1953, 1 November 1955, 14 November 1958, and 3 March 1964.

3. Randy Lovelace was made a full partner in late 1946 by his uncles, but I have been unable to uncover any details regarding that understanding.

up the nonprofit foundation, including the close liaison with Mayo, came to fruition on 24 September 1947 with the formal incorporation of the Lovelace Foundation for Medical Education and Research. Fourteen incorporators, including five physicians and nine laymen from New Mexico and around the country (see pp. 75–82) formed "a non-profit corporation without capital stock for educational, scientific, benevolent, and charitable purposes under the laws of the State of New Mexico." In the incorporation papers, eight specific objectives were laid out for the new foundation; five were more broad, while three contained a narrower focus. In the words of the charter, the foundation was intended

> to aid, engage in, conduct and foster in the broadest and most liberal manner medical, surgical, and scientific research and investigation and to apply the knowledge therefrom to the causes, prevention, relief and therapy of human diseases and to the benefit of mankind in general; . . . to initiate and further activities designed to promote public health; to provide instruction for practicing physicians and surgeons; to promote the education, training, skill, and investigative ability of physicians, scientists, and individuals engaged in work in the basic sciences which bear on medicine and surgery . . .[4]

To this general commitment to medical education and research were added three more specific objectives:

> to carry out basic and applied research in aviation medicine and in matters directly or indirectly related thereto; . . . to investigate and study the effect on health of residence in the southwestern part of the United States, and particularly in a dry climate; and to publish or assist in publishing the results of scientific investigations and observations made by members of the staff of the Lovelace Clinic and by persons connected with this foundation.[5]

4. Certificate of Incorporation, Lovelace Foundation for Medical Education and Research, 24 September 1947, in Lovelace Medical Foundation archives.

5. Ibid.

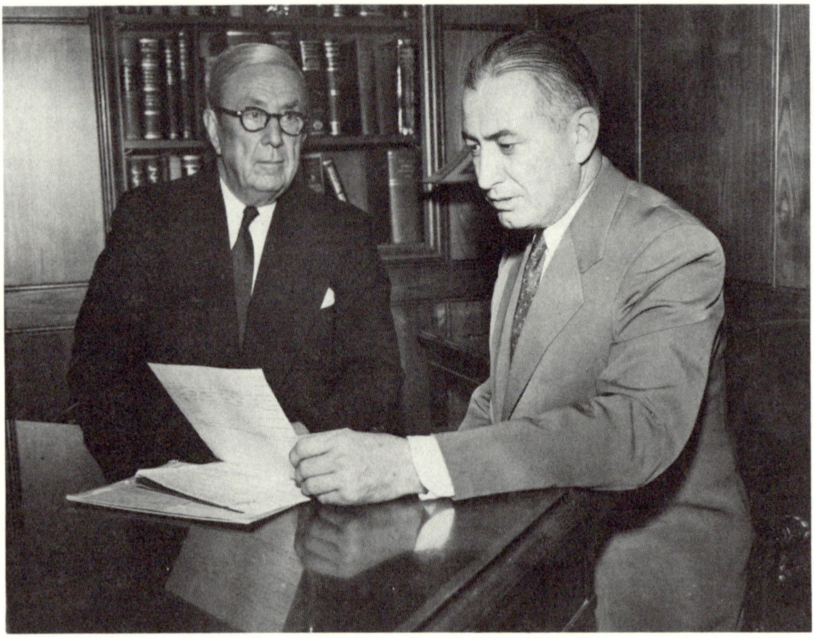

The two Drs. Lovelace look over the charter documents of the Lovelace Foundation, September, 1947.

These goals clearly reflected the medical and scholarly interests of Drs. Lovelace II (aviation medicine) and Lovelace I (climate in the therapy of tuberculosis and other diseases) as well as the practical problem of communicating with the rest of the scientific world from so relatively isolated and obscure a place as Albuquerque.

To provide a basic endowment for the new foundation, the three partners of the Lovelace Clinic agreed to donate that institution—which had seen more than twenty thousand patients during the preceding year—entirely to the new entity. The title, all equipment and miscellaneous property, accounts receivable, clinical records, library, and goodwill of the clinic were conveyed to the foundation through an irrevocable agreement of the two Drs. Lovelace and Dr. Lassetter. No precise value was placed on those assets, but they were conservatively estimated at over one million dollars, which was a considerable sum for the 1940s. But the contribution of the founders actually exceeded that sum by a wide margin. Randy Lovelace's plans for the future of the Lovelace Center explicitly called for more space (for more doctors, laboratory facilities, and so forth), and his Uncle Doc had already also agreed to help financially with that part of the plan. Within a year after the formation of the foundation, construction was underway for a new clinic-foundation building, on land donated for the purpose by Dr. Lovelace I—along with 125,000 dollars toward the cost of constructing the building itself. The assets of the clinic were all that the foundation possessed at its start, but its founders and supporters expected profits from the clinic's operation to provide working capital for future operations, liberally supplemented by other donations and contracts.

The structure of the clinic was also changed during the fall 1947 reformation. From a partnership controlled by its owners, there developed a voluntary association of salaried physicians, which operated under a board of governors and owned no property. The former partners of the clinic became salaried physicians like the other fifteen signatories of the original Articles of Association; in fact, of course, they continued to wield a very special influence. For example, both Drs. Lovelace were declared Associates for life under the terms of the association's original charter, and each held permanent positions on the clinic's Board of Governors. It was always clear that in the Lovelace Clinic the two Drs. Lovelace were first among equals.[6]

It was immediately evident to everyone associated with the new foundation that its prospects for success would depend, to a large degree, on the support and assistance afforded by its Board of Trustees. In selecting the original fourteen trustees, the founders sought to strike a judicious balance between New Mexicans and national figures and between physicians and nonphysicians. The first board included nine New Mexicans and five people from out of state. The New Mexico group had a strong nucleus of clinic doctors, including the two Drs. Love-

6. One longtime staffer who joined the clinic group in the early 1960s called the Lovelace operation "a benevolent despotism" at the time that he first observed it. Dr. Robert S. Turner, interview with the author, Albuquerque, 31 March 1986.

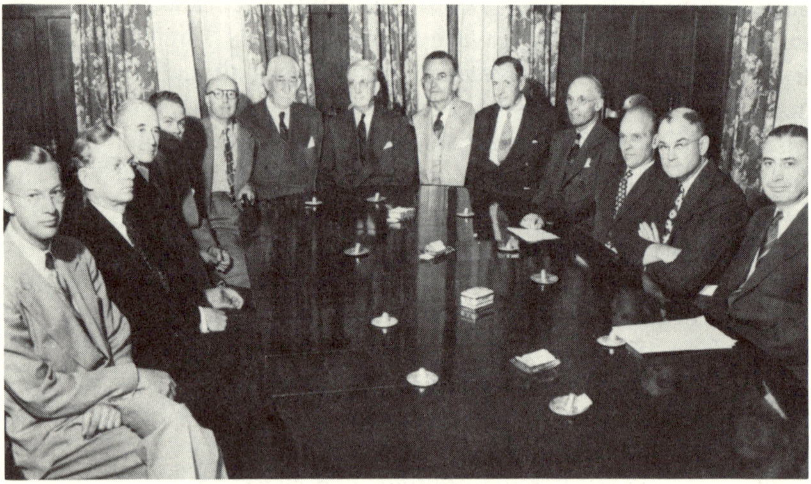

The original Board of Trustees of the Lovelace Foundation for Medical Education and Research at its first, formal meeting in September, 1947. Left to right: Dr. D. Angus McKinnon; Judge Sam Bratton; Cale Carson; Thomas Fortune Ryan III; Floyd Odlum; Dr. Edgar Lassetter; Dr. William Randolph Lovelace I; Oscar Love; Nelson Talbott; Albert Mitchell; Jack Korber; Dr. Ward Darley; and Dr. William Randolph Lovelace II.

lace and Dr. Lassetter as well as one member of the group of physicians who had joined the clinic in 1941, the young surgeon Dr. D. Angus McKinnon, Jr. Dr. McKinnon had formed a friendship with Randy Lovelace at the Mayo Clinic, and his abilities as a surgeon and his all-around good judgment had also quickly won Uncle Doc's confidence.[7] With the physicians on the board were five New Mexico laymen, each prominent in the civic and/or business affairs of the state, and including, for example, two Albuquerque bankers, Cale W. Carson, Sr., president of the city's First National Bank, and Oscar M. Love, cofounder and president of Albuquerque National Bank. Given their strategic positions within the New Mexico business community, the

7. Dr. McKinnon, the last survivor of that original Board of Trustees, lives in retirement in Albuquerque and still interests himself in the institution that he helped to found forty years ago. Dr. D. Angus McKinnon, Jr., interview with the author, Albuquerque, 25 October 1984.

bankers' help and support were central to the success of the new enterprise, and both of them were active, committed members of the board. Oscar Love, a longtime friend and patient of Uncle Doc Lovelace, was especially devoted to the institution and gave unstintingly of his time, good judgment, and resources.[8] An Albuquerque lawyer, Judge Sam G. Bratton of the U.S. Circuit Court, another old friend and ally of Dr. Lovelace I, was also one of the original incorporators of the foundation. A former U.S. senator and a prominent figure in state legal and political circles, Judge Bratton gave the Lovelace Medical Foundation valuable assistance before his death in 1963. Albuquerque businessman Jack Korber was a fourth nonphysician member of the original board. Korber was a successful and influential wholesaler with extensive business and personal ties throughout the region, and he was particularly close to the operations of the foundation during its early, tentative years.

The ninth New Mexico board member, and the only non-Albuquerquean of the group, was Albert Mitchell, who contributed enormously to the infant institution despite his physical distance from the place. (His home was on his Albert, New Mexico, ranch located on the plains of northeastern New Mexico; but Mitchell was a private pilot—one of the interests that linked him to Randy Lovelace—and he was a frequent visitor to the Lovelace medical complex.) A rancher and investor of considerable wealth, Mitchell gave generously of his own resources to help the foundation reach its goals—100,000 dollars to help in financing the completion of the clinic-foundation building; 30,000 dollars to equip a badly needed machine shop; 15,000 dollars here and 25,000 dollars there—but, just as importantly, he contributed his time and good counsel. Particularly significant was his influence in gaining entry for foundation personnel to places otherwise unreachable; for Mitchell had many friends and associates in high places in the worlds of government, business, and finance.[9] He served as vice chair-

8. Dr. Donald E. Kilgore, interview with the author, Albuquerque, 25 November 1985. Oscar Love's son, O. Mahlon Love, Jr., continues the Love family tradition of service to Lovelace. He has been a member of the foundation's board since 1972.

9. Ibid.

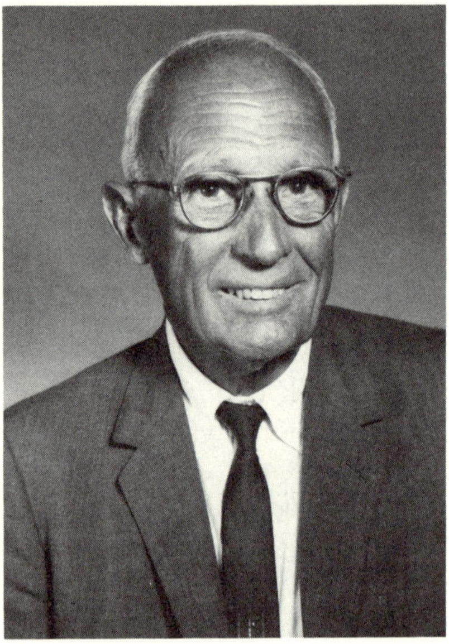

Albert Mitchell, long-time friend and supporter of the Lovelace medical center.

man of the foundation for many years, retiring from active service in 1972.

Although the roster of the Lovelace Foundation's Board of Trustees emphasized the New Mexico character of the enterprise, the New Mexican board members were joined by a small but influential group of non-natives. Chief among the national figures who agreed to give their aid and support to the Albuquerque institution was a relatively little known but powerful figure of corporate America named Floyd Odlum. A lawyer by training, Odlum had become a self-made millionaire during the Depression years, reorganizing companies in almost every type of industry, including banking, railroads, department stores, public utilities, motion pictures, aircraft, oil, and mining. His deals had led him into control of such diverse enterprises as the Greyhound bus line, the R.K.O. and Paramount motion-picture studios, the Hilton hotel chain, the Bonwit Teller and Franklin Simon retail chains, uranium mines, and an occasional bank or oil company.[10] In addition, he played a major part in

10. For sketches of Odlum's career, see *The National Cyclopedia of American Biography,* Current Volume F (1939–42), pp. 476–77; "Floyd Odlum and the Work Ethic," *New York Times,* 28 January 1973; and his obituary, *New York Times,* 18 June 1976.

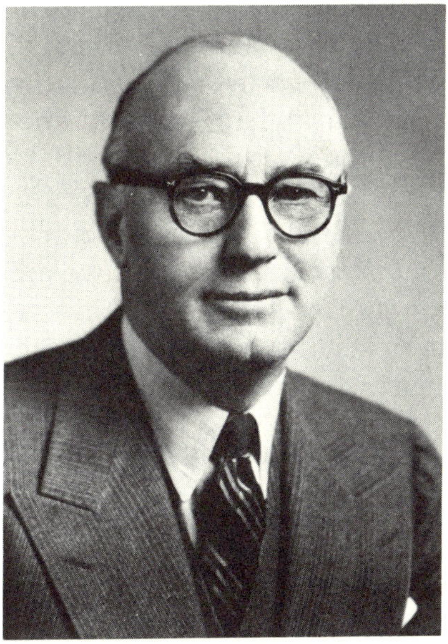

Floyd Odlum, chairman of the Lovelace Foundation's board, 1947–1967.

the nation's public life as director of the Office of Production Management during World War Two and as an advocate of the development of the Atlas missile, which started humanity on its way to the moon.

Odlum became interested in the Albuquerque experiment through Randy Lovelace, whom he met at the Mayo Clinic in 1937. Randy was one of his physicians there, and Odlum quickly came to respect his surgical skills and his obvious commitment to the best in patient care. But the relationship was enormously intensified by the men's mutual interest in aviation. Odlum had received his first exposure to the world of corporate aviation when his Atlas Corporation took control of Curtiss-Wright Corporation in the late 1920s, but it was his 1936 marriage to aviatrix Jacqueline Cochran that drew him closer to the industry. Through her, he became interested in high performance aircraft, flight records and speed, and the stress on humans of flight at high speeds or altitudes; and this personal contact helped to trigger an increasingly heavy professional interest in the world of flight during the 1940s. He bought controlling interest in Northeast Airlines in 1943, and four years later he gained control of Consolidated Vultee Aircraft Corporation, or Convair. Odlum and Randy Lovelace both spoke the language of aviation, and the financier was also attracted by the young Albuquerque surgeon's charm, personal dynamism, and special expertise. In short order, Randy grew close personally to both Odlum and his wife. Given the influence and power the financier wielded, especially in the airline and aircraft industries, Odlum was a natural for membership on the Lovelace Foundation board and an obvious choice as its first chairman. In fact, Odlum also already knew something about the prospects and problems of medical research. He was founder and honorary national chairman of the Arthritis and Rheumatism Foundation—he suffered terribly from crippling arthritis—and that experience provided him with a special awareness and sensitivity to the subject.

For twenty years, until his retirement in 1967, Floyd Odlum served ably as chairman of the Lovelace Foundation. (He was chairman emeritus thereafter, and remained close to the work in Albuquerque until his death in 1976.) He was an active chairman, keeping well informed on developments in Albuquerque, although he was content to leave the day-to-day control of operations in the hands of people on the scene. He supported the foundation with his money, but he was perhaps even more important in enlisting his colleagues from high finance to support the experiment in Albuquerque. For example, it was largely through his influence that John Hertz, founder of the Yellow Cab Company, Hertz Drive-Ur-Self Corporation, and much else, came to the assistance of the Lovelace Foundation. (Hertz served actively on its Board of Trustees until his death in 1961, giving solid support to the foundation's endeavors.) The same was true for John Jay Hopkins, one of the major figures of American finance and industry at midcentury. Hopkins, president and chairman of the board of General Dynamics Corporation, contributed generously and worked hard for the Lovelace Foundation as an active member of its board until his death in 1957. He personally provided much of the funding to establish the Radiation Therapy Center at Lovelace, and he enthusiastically encouraged the foundation's involvement in the then infant field of nuclear medicine. Ellsworth Alvord, a corporate attorney specializing in tax matters and one of the nation's premier experts in that field, was another personal friend and adviser to Odlum who, through him, became involved with the Lovelace Foundation. (When the foundation confronted serious problems with the Internal Revenue Service regarding its tax status in the early 1950s, it was Alvord who resolved the difficulty.) David G. Baird, financier and insurance magnate, was another Odlum associate who helped the Lovelace pioneers during the early, critical years of their work. Although there is no indication that he ever set foot in Albuquerque, he contributed generously—well into six-figure sums—to help the clinic-foundation with its building program in the early 1950s. The list could be extended, further corroborating the fact that Floyd Odlum's personal service and his recruitment of his friends and associates—some of whom, like Baird, had little or no other contact with the place—proved to be of inestimable value to the Lovelace Foundation during its formative years.

In addition to the Odlum colleagues, other "outsiders" played important roles, particularly in the foundation's early years. Dr. Ward Darley, dean of the University of Colorado Medical School and later executive director of the Association of American Medical Colleges, was one of the original fourteen incorporators of the foundation and helped in establishing its educational planning and contacts. Randy Lovelace directly recruited the other two members of the first Board of Trustees—Thomas Fortune Ryan III, scion of the New York railroad and banking family, and Nelson S. Talbott, a Dayton, Ohio, businessman involved in several spheres of the aviation industry. Randy met and became friends with both Ryan and Talbott in the late 1930s and early 1940s. Their common interest in aviation was their major bond. In the later 1940s, Ryan was a director and chairman of the board of Mid-Continental Airlines, and Talbott was active on the board of directors of Trans World Airlines. The presence on the Lovelace board of so many eminent names from the world of aviation—Odlum, Hopkins, Ryan, and Talbott among them—was consistent with the foundation's stated interest in aviation medicine; and aviation people remained prominent and active in support of the institution throughout the first thirty years or more of its existence. Other prominent outsiders who furnished the foundation with strong support included C. R. Smith, longtime president of American Airlines, who gave twenty-four years of active service on the Lovelace board; Earl D. Johnson, president of General Dynamics and vice president of Delta Airlines (and a member of the board for more than twenty years); and William P. "Bill" Lear, the electrical engineering genius whose Lear Jet Corporation has played so prominent a role in civilian aircraft design and manufacture, and others. Smith and Johnson in particular, were both close personal friends of Randy Lovelace, and they remained strong allies and boosters of the foundation and clinic, with each man preserving his commitment to the Albuquerque center for more than thirty years.

These busy and talented men were on the original Board of Trustees for the Lovelace Foundation, but there were others who contributed importantly to the foundation's success during the first two decades of its existence. New Mexico rancher and businessman E. T. Springer; Senator Clinton P. Anderson and his son Sherburne; university president (Stanford University and State University of New York) and educational consultant Alvin Eurich; Albuquerque accountant and counselor J. Bryan Stephenson; and others were helpful trustees or friends who played active parts in the institution's history during its first two decades. One special person who joined the board in 1962, and whose influence rose steadily thereafter, was New Mexico oilman, rancher, and businessman Robert O. Anderson. Attracted to support the foundation by Randy Lovelace, again, Anderson succeeded Floyd Odlum in 1967 as chairman of the board, and played an even more important role in the institution's second twenty years than Odlum had done in the beginning.[11]

While a strong board was necessary for the success of Albuquerque's new Lovelace Center, the clinic was clearly the indispensable cornerstone of the whole operation, at least for

11. See pp. 154–159 and *passim* for a more thorough discussion of Anderson's service to the Albuquerque medical center.

its foreseeable future. In 1947, the clinic was a reasonable starting point for the kind of institution that Randy Lovelace envisioned, but it was no more than simply a beginning. It was a strong regional institution with an honorable reputation, but it lacked significant financial resources and could hardly be thought of as some kind of money machine from which revenues to fund extensive foundation operations could be obtained. Its doctors were well-trained, highly regarded physicians representing roughly a half-dozen major medical specialties, and the Lovelace Clinic was in good position to play a major role in the development of medicine in postwar New Mexico. It was an institution a country doctor, like Uncle Doc Lovelace, could be proud of, but Randy Lovelace's dream was bigger. He thought in terms of a large, nationally prominent clinic—perhaps not so large and influential as the Mayo Clinic or the Cleveland Clinic, but definitely an institution of that class.[12] In 1947, there was an acute need to emphasize the clinic and to promote its expansion as rapidly as possible if the clinic were to fulfill its role of carrying the entire operation, at least to large degree, through the early years. Thus, an aggressive and quick expansion of Uncle Doc's clinic was high on Randy Lovelace's agenda.

Inherent in that expansion was a large-scale physical enlargement of the clinic to provide space for new physicians and for the laboratories of the Lovelace Foundation research personnel and interested clinicians. The notion of expanding within the downtown bank building was considered briefly, then abandoned because of its impracticality and prohibitive expense. Consideration was given next to the purchase and renovation of the building and property of the old Sandia Girls' School, located on Gibson Boulevard near Carlisle Southeast. (The building still stands as the Kirtland Officers' Club, West.) Uncle

12. There were those who smirked at the dimensions of his imagination in the late forties, but less than ten years later, when the nation's major clinics or group practices organized themselves for purposes of consultation into a so-called Big Six association, the original six were the Mayo Clinic, Boston's Lahey Clinic, the Cleveland Clinic, Ochsner Clinic in New Orleans, the Henry Ford Hospital in Detroit, . . . and the Lovelace Clinic.

Doc took an option on the property and the foundation tried to work out a deal for the site, but for various reasons the plan fell through.[13] Attention then turned to land owned by Uncle Doc between Gibson Boulevard and Ridgecrest Drive in the city's southeast heights, a triangular tract of land encompassing approximately forty acres. This property had much to recommend it. In the first place, it was "in hand," and Dr. Lovelace I was prepared to donate whatever part of it the foundation might need, thus saving land-acquisition costs and making possible more building. Second, the land, stretching from San Mateo Boulevard in the west to Louisiana Boulevard in the east, was immediately adjacent to the air force base; indeed, it was bounded by base property on two of its three edges. (Additionally, the Albuquerque municipal airport was a mile or so west of the property in question, and merged with the air base.) Given the close relationship that Randy Lovelace anticipated between the foundation and the aviation industry, in general, and the air force, in particular, the physical proximity of the Lovelace Foundation to the air base and airport was highly desirable and might be especially advantageous. The property was also adjacent to the Veterans' Administration Hospital in Albuquerque, a juxtaposition that appeared particularly attractive in the late forties. In 1946 federal authorities had just completed construction of a large 250-bed new wing on their Albuquerque campus, and that facility figured in VA plans for the future as *the* military center for tuberculosis treatment. Thus, in 1947 it appeared likely that the VA Hospital was on the brink of emerging as the center of medical activity in the city, and the Lovelace Medical Center might benefit from close proximity to it.

There were worries, of course, about the Gibson site. In the late 1940s, Gibson Boulevard was well outside the central core of the city, and indeed was somewhat isolated out on the southeast mesa. It was particularly far from downtown Albuquerque, then still the hub of the city, and was poorly served by public

13. Dr. Clayton S. White, interview with the author, Albuquerque, 14 October 1985; George Savage, interview with the author, 28 January 1985; and Lovelace Medical Foundation, Board of Trustees, Minutes, 21 July 1948.

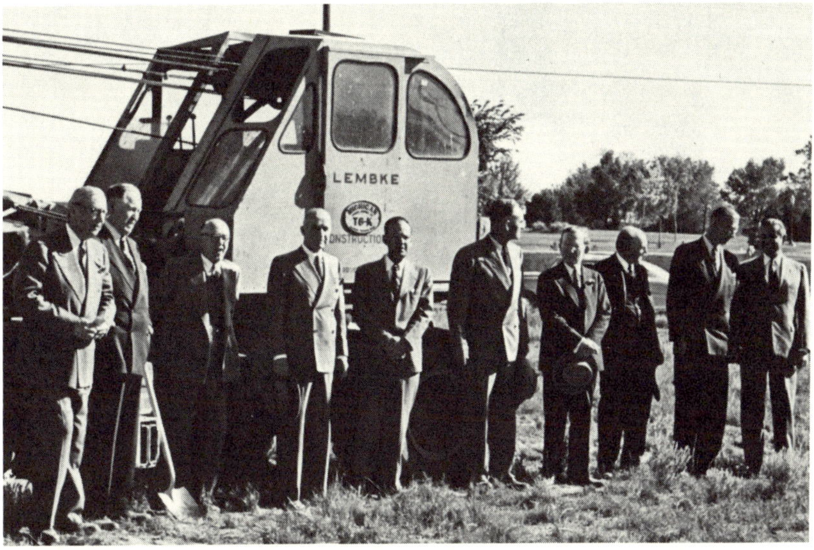

Groundbreaking ceremonies for the new Lovelace Clinic building, August, 1949. Left to right: Dr. William Randolph Lovelace I; Governor of New Mexico Thomas J. Mabry; Floyd Odlum; Cale Carson; unidentified; Oscar Love; Sam Bratton; architect John Gaw Meem; Dr. D. Angus McKinnon; Dr. Randy Lovelace.

transportation. And it was outside the most rapidly developing quadrants of the city, most notably the northeast heights. Also of some concern was the fact that Uncle Doc's proffered tract on Gibson presented only one face to the outside world, bounded as it was on two of its three sides by federal reservation land.[14]

At a special Board of Trustees meeting called in July 1948 explicitly for the purpose of discussing the space problem and its possible solution, it was agreed to make one final effort to obtain the Sandia School property and, failing that, to build a new clinic-foundation building on the Gibson site next to the VA Hospital and air base.[15] Renewed efforts to buy the school

14. In later years, these location problems became acutely apparent to the Lovelace institution. In the 1950s, 1960s, and 1970s, the city grew away from Lovelace, expanding vigorously to the northeast and north, and finally to the west; and the site of the Lovelace Foundation on the southeastern edge of the city proved to be a real handicap to both the clinic and the foundation's hospital.

15. Lovelace Medical Foundation, Board of Trustees, Minutes, 21 July 1948.

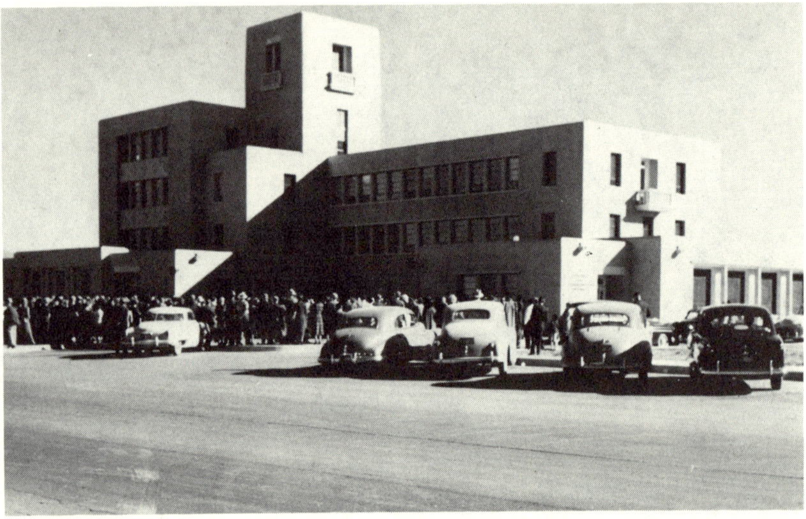

Crowd gathered before the new Lovelace Clinic building on Gibson Boulevard at its dedication in October, 1950.

property failed, and the new foundation turned to the task of building from scratch. Preliminary planning for this last contingency had already taken place, for Randy had requested tentative plans for a new clinic building from the St. Paul Minnesota architectural consulting firm Ellerby and Company, which was, not coincidentally, the firm responsible for much of the construction at the Mayo Clinic. However, most of the work in designing the new building, certainly its exterior, would be entrusted to an old friend and patient of Dr. Lovelace I, John Gaw Meem of Santa Fe. Meem was another of the old "lungers" who had come to New Mexico during the first decades of the twentieth century, seeking relief from a chest malady. By the late 1940s he had established a name for his pueblo-style architecture, and several of his buildings—most notably Santa Fe's School of American Research, Santa Fe's La Fonda Hotel, and several major buildings on the University of New Mexico campus—had already or would shortly attract national attention. The Lovelace planners intended their building to fit within the revivalist movement led by Meem, and the Santa Fean agreed to try to blend his traditional style architecture with the needs of a modern, twentieth-century medical clinic.

The building that Meem produced is one of the finest examples of his work. Construction started in the fall of 1949, and the fifty-thousand square-foot structure was ready for occupancy in October 1950. (At its grand opening ceremonies, Dr. Charles Mayo was, appropriately, the chief speaker.) It comfortably housed the clinic's twenty-nine physicians and the foundation's still tiny research staff, with ample room left over for expansion. For the next thirty-five years, the Clinic Building, or Building 1—the names by which it has always been known—remained the heart of the Lovelace Clinic. Enlarged and remodeled several times over the years, it has consistently housed the majority of the staff's clinicians, concentrating, as group practices were supposed to do, a large repository of clinical expertise in one single place. Only a year after its occupancy, construction began on a new 20,000 square-foot wing, known as the Baird Wing, and the finished structure was ready for use in the fall of 1952.[16] This addition was intended primarily as laboratory space which would free more footage in the original building for clinical purposes, but the Baird Wing has also been used as clinical space over the years. Then, in November 1953, a 7,500 square-foot Radiation Therapy Center was opened, adding to the clinic's treatment capabilities; and in July 1961, a 5,000 square-foot OB-Gyn Building was constructed. All told, in just over a decade the Lovelace Foundation developed facilities, totaling around 80,000 square feet of space, which were used predominantly by the Lovelace Clinic for clinical purposes. (Two other major construction projects—totaling 155,000 square feet of space, and used largely for research and administrative purposes—will be mentioned presently.) Such a large physical plant was essential because during the same time frame the staff of the clinic increased 250 percent, from twenty-three doctors in 1950 to fifty-nine in 1962.

Table 1 traces the remarkable growth of the Lovelace Clinic during the brief period from its reorganization in 1947 until Randy Lovelace's death in 1965. From the dozen or so staff members at the start of 1947, the clinic's physicians increased

16. The addition was named to honor trustee David Baird who funded the work through the Lansing Foundation. Total cost of the addition exceeded 350,000 dollars.

Table 1 Lovelace Clinic Staff, 1941–1965

Year	*No. of MDs*	*Year*	*No. of MDs*
1941	12	1954	30
1942	14	1955	30
1943	18*	1956	41
1944	18*	1957	41
1945	15*	1958	43
1946	15*	1959	51
1947	16*	1960	46
1948	21	1961	55
1949	19	1962	59
1950	23	1963	64
1951	29	1964	68
1952	32	1965	75
1953	30		

*Includes staff members away in military service and temporary staffers.
These figures do not include MDs and PhDs on the Lovelace Foundation staff.

to seventy-five at the end of 1965. Of course, these mushrooming figures also reflect a large increase in clinic business, with 20,000 patient visits in 1947 to more than 177,000 in 1965. Part of the expansion in the number of physicians was simply a matter of adding new staffers in departments where patient loads were heaviest. For example, the clinic's staff listed only three internists in 1947, with other staff members—such as Dr. Clayton S. "Sam" White (see pp. 104–106), soon to be named research director for the foundation—filling in around the edges. By 1965, however, the number of internists had risen to twenty-five, including most of the major subspecialties within the discipline. Much the same could be said for orthopedic surgery, which Dr. Lew Overton performed alone in 1947, but by 1965 was joined by four other colleagues.

In addition to the obvious numerical expansion during that era, there was further differentiation within the staff. The new Lovelace Clinic of the 1950s and 1960s continued the tradition, begun by Uncle Doc's clinic in the late 1920s and 1930s, of adding people representing new fields and subspecializations as quickly as they developed. The dozen physicians of the clinic's staff in early 1947 represented six specialty fields—internal medicine, general surgery, pediatrics, radiology, obstetrics and gynecology, and chest medicine—but almost annually thereafter, new specialties were added, greatly increasing the range of services offered by the staff. An orthopedic surgeon joined the group in 1947—Lew Overton, a Mayo-trained surgeon who gave twenty-five years of distinguished service to the clinic and to New Mexico medicine in general—along with board-certified men in ophthalmology and aviation medicine. In the next year, a thoracic surgeon (Dr. Rodger MacQuigg) and a urologist were added, and in 1949 a pathologist and rheumatologist (Dr. Clarence M. "Bud" Kemper) joined the group. The clinic's first psychiatrist, dermatologist, and plastic surgeon came in 1950. Three short years after the 1947 reorganization of the Lovelace Clinic, its staff had grown from twelve physicians representing six specialty fields to nearly thirty doctors spanning some sixteen areas. By the time of Randy Lovelace's death in 1965, the seventy-five physicians of the clinic staff included board-certified specialists from two dozen fields, and many of them were the first or among the first to offer their particular expertise in New Mexico. Albuquerque was still "a general practice town" in the early postwar era,[17] with some conspicuous exceptions, but a radical change toward specialty medicine took place in the late 1940s and 1950s, and the Lovelace Clinic played a major part in that process.

There were stresses and strains associated with such growth. For one thing, the distance between the group practitioners of the Lovelace Clinic and the downtown doctors tended to grow rather than diminish during this period. To the unhappy tradition of mistrust, suspicion, and dislike inherited from the 1930s were added the special heat produced by increased economic competition and the anxiety inherent in the rapidly changing times. Newcomers arriving in town—both clinic men and solo practitioners—immediately grew aware of the strong polarization in the community, and the level of competition was multiplied by the ambitious expansion and plans of the

17. Dr. Albert G. Simms III, interview with the author, Albuquerque, 17 May 1984.

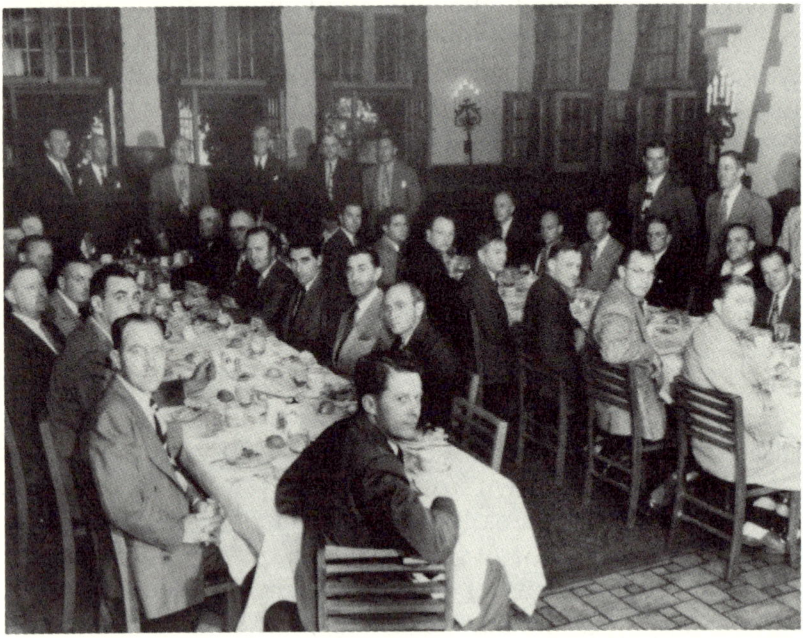

Lovelace Clinic staff members and members of the Lovelace Foundation's Board of Trustees at a formal banquet in the late forties.

clinic after 1947. The construction of the new Lovelace Clinic building in 1950 and the opening of Bataan Memorial Methodist Hospital—"the clinic's hospital"—two years later (see pp. 93–98) broadened the split by physically removing the clinic's doctors from most of the everyday activity of the town's medical community in the hallways of the First National Bank building and the downtown hospitals; however, the physical separation of the two camps was by no means complete.[18]

Regrettably, the local medical society did little to smooth relations among the town's doctors. In fact, it could well be

18 Dr. Robert Massey stressed the importance of the physical isolation of the clinic's staff in their facilities on the southeastern periphery of the city and the inevitable loss of interaction and communication with the rest of the town's physicians. He also contributed the interesting idea that the creation of a medical school by the University of New Mexico in the early 1960s had the side effect of pulling the hostile groups together in a common enterprise, providing a meeting place, as it were, for the rival elements. Dr. Robert U. Massey, interview with the author, Farmington, Conn., 4 January 1985.

argued that the Bernalillo County Medical Association was a participant far too often in the quarreling, rather than acting as a neutral instrument of mediation. The grievance procedures of the county society were regularly used to chastise or to threaten the clinic, most often on charges of "advertising." This disquiet within the Albuquerque medical community was usually concealed, but the tension and suspicion associated with the clinic's leap forward in the late 1940s and early 1950s brought a nasty public display in 1952. In that year, serious charges were presented to the grievance committee of the county society, alleging once again unethical advertising by the clinic. The protest was occasioned by a series of articles, appearing in newspapers across the country, written by the nationally syndicated columnist Robert Ruark. The articles—effusively titled, for example, "Medicine at Its Best" (*Los Angeles Daily News*, 6 May 1952) and "Selfless Doctors" (*New York World Telegram*, 30 April 1952)—hymned the praises of the progressive new medical center created by the Lovelaces, and by implication they scorned, or at least questioned, the competency of Albuquerque's nonclinic physicians.[19] A petition demanding censure of the clinic and its physicians was quickly drafted and eventually signed by more than fifty community doctors, and the grievance committee of the county medical association requested a formal answer from the clinic to the charges. The incident eventually blew over, as did many other less heated episodes of the sort, but not before tense committee meetings and a great deal of private, bitter grousing and gossiping had widened the breach between the Lovelace group and the city's other doctors.[20]

19. One of the several longtime Albuquerque practitioners who talked to me about this incident was a doctor who was close to the center of the downtown doctors' camp. He recalled a phrase alluding to "the downtown hackers" as appearing in the Ruark articles. Neither that phrase nor anything similar actually appeared in the articles, but his recollection suggests the impression (and anger) of the downtown doctors at the time. Another of the anti-clinic faction told me of a colleague who bitterly kept an actual count and record of the number of times that reference to Randy Lovelace's parachute jump showed up in the local papers. Private communications.

20. Ruark himself was dragged into this unedifying squabble and wrote an angry letter to the Bernalillo County Medical Association, denying that anyone at the Lovelace Clinic had encouraged or helped him to write the articles, "it being a point of special pride with me that no one has ever been able to *get* me to write anything." Robert Ruark to Bernalillo County Medical Society, 11 October 1952, in Lovelace Medical Foundation archives.

One of the legacies of this particular early 1950s incident was the firm identification many Lovelace clinicians made of the county medical society as "the enemy," a label that was accurate according to considerable evidence. Frequent complaints found in Lovelace Clinic staff documents as well as recollections by Lovelace veterans of the fifties and sixties regarding the county association's hostility toward Lovelace and their exclusion from its positions of leadership underscore the point.[21] The relationship reached an absolute nadir in 1973, when a majority of the clinic staff voted to secede entirely from the Bernalillo County group and to form their own, separate society linked directly to the state organization.[22] This proposal, calling for the formation of the Sandia Medical Society, quickly died, but the incident demonstrates the dimensions of the estrangement between the Lovelace group and the corporate organization which supposedly represented it to the outside world. On the other hand, the state society was more remote and rarely involved (or consciously tried to remain distant) in the wranglings in Albuquerque. Lovelace physicians actually found a considerably warmer welcome and greater opportunity for participation in the state society than in their local one. One of the longtime leaders of the clinic staff, Dr. Lew Overton, was elected president of the New Mexico Medical Society in 1959-60; and one of the clinic's rheumatologists, Dr. Ronald V. Dorn, held numerous positions of responsibility within the state society throughout the 1950s and 1960s.[23]

21. Prior to 1961, the Lovelace Clinic, with approximately 25 percent of the BCMA membership and contributing approximately 25 percent of its support, had never had a member of its staff elected to the Board of Governors panel which ran the county association. The election of clinic pediatrician Dr. Roy Goddard in the fall of that year finally broke the pattern.

22. Lovelace Clinic, Board of Governors, Minutes, 9 January 1973.

23. Neither of the Drs. Lovelace was ever honored by election to high office within the local or state societies after Dr. Lovelace I's election to the presidency of the Bernalillo County Medical Association in 1916. One of the ironic fruits of the bitter professional politics in Albuquerque was the fact that Uncle Doc Lovelace could win election as president of the United States Section of the International College of Surgeons (1956), and Randy Lovelace could establish an international reputation in the worlds of medicine and medical research, yet neither was honored in that way by their local peers.

One of the major developments in the early history of the reorganized Lovelace operation was the opening in April 1952 of the new 104-bed Bataan Memorial Methodist Hospital on land immediately adjacent to the one-year-old Lovelace Clinic building. As the population of Albuquerque and the surrounding area began to escalate in the immediate postwar era, the region found itself confronted with a serious hospital bed shortage. Still operating in the city were a number of the old sanatoria dedicated to the care of tuberculosis patients, but the arrival of streptomycin and other modern drugs that were effective against that disease were quickly making this institution a medical anachronism; few sanatoria made the transition into the new era.[24] While beds were lying vacant in the sanatoria, general hospital beds were increasingly at a premium in the rapidly growing city. In 1950 there was a total of 213 beds available for the 146,000 people of Bernalillo County, plus another 43,000 in the three immediately adjacent counties—1 bed for every 887 people.[25] With the region's population skyrocketing year by year, an acute crisis loomed on the horizon.

As early as 1912, the women of the Methodist Church first became involved in the provision of health services, specifically hospital care, in New Mexico. In that year, the Reverend Thomas Harwood, a pioneer Methodist missionary in the territory, deeded two acres of land to a group of Methodist churchwomen for the purpose of establishing a sanatorium to help in caring for the tuberculars then flooding the region. These women enlisted the help of the Women's Home Missionary Society of the national Methodist Church, and this external support, together with the Harwood land and other donations, made possible the opening of the Methodist Deaconess Sanatorium in 1912. The new facility was primitive, originally consisting of four tents and a seven-room house, and it had space to care for

24. Presbyterian Hospital and St. Joseph Hospital, both of which started as tuberculosis sanatoria, are conspicuous exceptions.

25. For comparative purposes, in 1985 there were 1,559 short-term, nonfederal hospital beds available to the 466,000 people of Bernalillo County alone, or a ratio of 1 bed for every 299 people. Health Resources Registry, University of New Mexico School of Medicine.

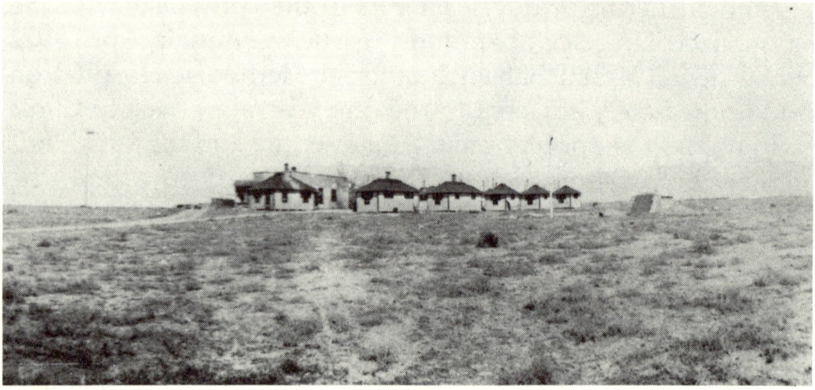

The Methodist Deaconess Sanatorium, predecessor to Bataan Memorial Methodist Hospital, as it looked between 1912 and 1916.

sixteen patients. (In the 1930s, when the institution reached its maximum size, it housed sixty-five patients.) Located on East Central Avenue, at approximately the present-day intersection of Central Avenue and University Boulevard, it was one of several sanatoria to be found on that street, which was then dubbed "San Alley." When fully developed, the Methodist institution consisted of three main buildings plus a number of cottages designed to allow the patients to capitalize on the fresh, bracing air of the region. For thirty-eight years it served the lung-sick pilgrims who sought a new lease on life in the mountain West. By the end of the 1940s, however, the days of the old tuberculosis sanatoria were clearly numbered, and the physical plant on Central Avenue did not seem to be a good candidate for conversion to general hospital use. In the spring and summer of 1949, it was decided to sell that property and to use the money received as a nucleus for building a new community hospital.

Planning for the new hospital received a powerful impetus when Dr. Lovelace I offered to donate land for the institution adjacent to the site of the new Lovelace Clinic building. He was a member of the Methodist Church—though not a particularly active one—and the opportunity to participate in this worthy church project undoubtedly appealed to him. Far more important, however, was the obvious advantage of having a brand new general hospital in close proximity to his expanding clinic. Discussions with agents of the church quickly resulted in an agreement that, if the church accepted his land offer, the Methodist hospital would institute an open staff policy; but it was also at least tacitly understood that by the very geography of things (and by virtue of the special unity inherent in the clinic's organization) the staff of the Lovelace Clinic would inevitably enjoy a special voice within the affairs of the new hospital. Despite the "political" problems thus raised, the women of the Methodist Church, acting through their Women's Society of Christian Service, decided to accept Dr. Lovelace's offer and moved on to the task of raising money for their building project.

Early calculations indicated that construction of a 104-bed hospital, outfitted and equipped in the most up-to-date fashion, would require approximately 1.5 million dollars. Methodist Church national headquarters immediately pledged 450,000 dollars—essentially the sum derived from the sale of the Central Avenue property—and the remainder was to be raised locally through general popular subscription and by special appeal to members of the Methodist Church. A fundraising committee of powerful local lay leaders in the church was appointed in September 1949, and the work of raising the million dollars needed for the start of construction commenced. Two Lovelace Foundation trustees, Oscar Love and Albert Mitchell, were prominent on that committee. The fundraisers also included a future trustee, J. Bryan Stephenson; a Lovelace administrator, John Dornacker; Randy Lovelace's father-in-law, Earl Moulton; and several other close friends of the Lovelace endeavor. As individuals, "Lovelace people" participated actively in the fundraising for the new hospital; and both individually and corporatively, they made significant contributions to the project. In mid-1950 the campaign reached its objective, and construction of the new hospital started on 5 November 1950.[26]

26. The Methodist hospital, like the new Lovelace Clinic building west of it, was designed by John Gaw Meem, and it also represented his Southwest style at its finest. On groundbreaking day, participants and onlookers could look immediately west of the hospital site to get a good idea of what the structure would finally resemble. The Lovelace Clinic building had opened only two weeks before the hospital groundbreaking.

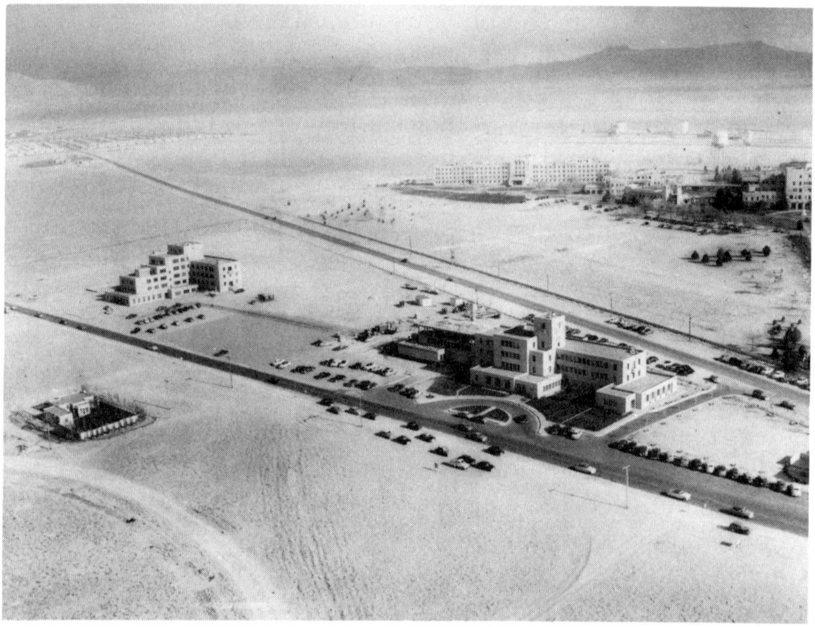

An aerial view of the Gibson Boulevard campus in 1952. The Lovelace Clinic building with the Baird Memorial Wing under construction is at the right, and the brand new Bataan Memorial Methodist Hospital is at the left. Across Ridgecrest Boulevard to the right rear stands the Veterans' Administration Hospital.

The new institution was ready by the spring of 1952. It was named Bataan Memorial Methodist Hospital as a living memorial to the New Mexico soldiers of the 200th Army Coast Artillery which had fought and suffered in the World War II battle for the Bataan Peninsula in the Philippines and the infamous death march associated with it. Formally opening its doors on 28 April 1952, it immediately began to play a major role in the health-care system of Albuquerque and the region at large. For example, its physical growth was fast and impressive, with a new wing constructed in 1959 bringing its capacity to 163 beds and with other additions and modifications increasing its size to 216 beds by 1963. (It reached its maximum size in 1966 with expansion to 245 beds.) Within a dozen years of its opening, it was admitting 8,500 patients per year.[27] Just as impressive as its sheer growth was its record of innovation, for a long list of "firsts" marks the history of the hospital during its first decades of service. In 1957, it opened the state's first intensive-care unit, and the first open heart surgery in New Mexico was performed at Bataan in 1959, as was the first kidney dialysis in the same year. The state's first Virus Laboratory and Radioisotope Laboratory (both in association with the Lovelace Foundation), thermogram capability, and exterior fetal heart monitor were all located at Bataan; and the list could well be extended. Especially noteworthy were the several national "firsts" recorded at Bataan, including the first American hospital with a heart-lung resuscitator and its distinction as the nation's first cystic fibrosis research and treatment center. It claimed two world-wide "firsts": Bataan Hospital created one of the world's first laminar flow "clean air" operating rooms in 1966, and the world's first lung lavage procedure to flush radioactive particles from a patient's lungs was performed within its walls in 1971. By the end of its second decade of service, the hospital had seen its 1952 budget of 520,000 dollars expand to over 6.8 million dollars, its original staff of physicians grow from 69 members to 278, and its professional nursing and ancillary staff expand from 112 to 542 in 1972.

Until 1965, Bataan operated under the auspices of the Women's Division of Christian Service of the Board of Missions of the Methodist Church, and functioned under the supervision of an advisory board composed of outstanding business and civic leaders throughout New Mexico. In 1965, ownership of the institution was shifted from the national church agency to the New Mexico Annual Conference of the Methodist Church, and Bataan became strictly a local institution. Not long afterward, in October 1969, Bataan Hospital was purchased by the Lovelace Medical Foundation (see pp. 156–159), and the church-sponsored hospital became a full, official part of the Lovelace family of institutions. From its very inception, however, it was

27. Of the 8,421 patients admitted to Bataan Hospital in 1964, 6,579 (78 percent) were admitted by physicians of the Lovelace Clinic. Bataan Memorial Hospital, *Annual Report, 1964*, 17 February 1965, attachment 2.

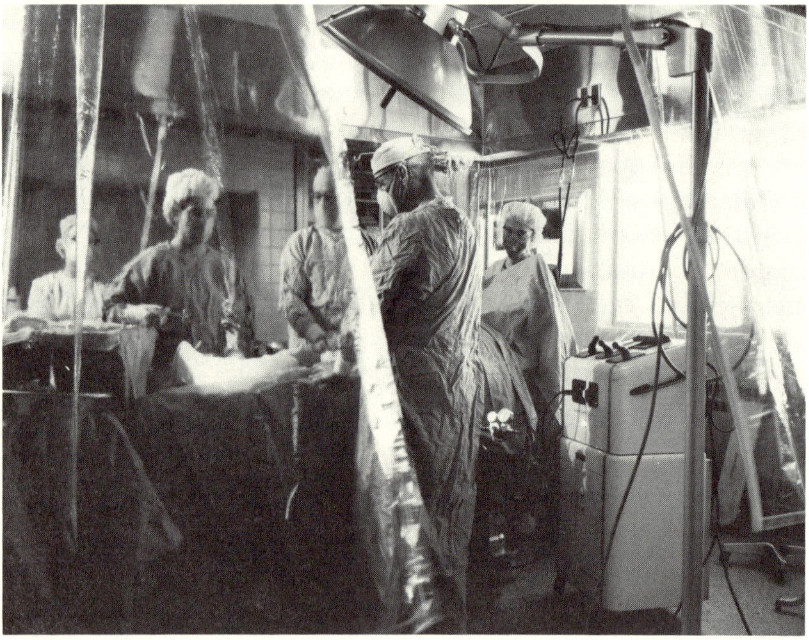

Bataan Hospital's innovative laminar flow operating room around 1966. The surgeon in the picture is Dr. Lew Overton, longtime head of the Lovelace Clinic's department of orthopaedic surgery.

an essential component in the success of the Lovelace dream in Albuquerque.

Internally, the years between 1947 and 1965 witnessed few changes of major dimensions at the Lovelace Clinic in terms of its organization and system of operation. Although it was in theory an association of physicians run by an elected Board of Governors, it was in fact a thinly veiled, though benign, autocracy. What had been Uncle Doc's clinic was Randy's operation during that period. It was Randy who was basically responsible for charting the institution's course, selecting its people, and fighting the fires that inevitably flared in an organization of such size and complexity. In the overall scheme of things, it was formally his position as director of the Lovelace Medical Foundation that conferred special authority on him, for the clinic was a kind of contractor to the foundation for the provision of medical services as well as the leasor of buildings and equipment from the foundation. Dr. Lovelace II was also a life member of the clinic's six-man Board of Governors, and in 1960 he became formally its vice chairman. (From 1947 until his death in 1968, Uncle Doc was chairman of the clinic's Board of Governors.) But still more of his authority stemmed quite naturally from the force of his personality and charm and, most importantly of all, from the unbroken chain of successes that the Lovelace operation enjoyed under his direction. He was not heavy handed in style, preferring to lead by persuasion and example, and always setting high personal standards of expectation and performance in his work. Yet, at the same time, there was no doubt about who was in charge, and he could be angry and obstinate on the rare occasions when ideas or plans he firmly believed in were seriously challenged or threatened. The full dimensions of his authority—and the resultant time demands on him—are well documented within the clinic's records and in the memories of those with whom he worked; and yet the "yoke" was a light one and easily borne. There was much of the natural diplomat in Randy Lovelace, and he far more often elicited cooperation than confrontation from those with whom he worked.

Throughout the period under discussion, the senior Dr. Lovelace continued to involve himself, if in reduced measure, in the affairs of the clinic that he had raised to stature. He aged gracefully and easily through his seventies and early eighties, with both his physical health and intellect remaining strong. He came to the clinic daily, and continued to see some of his old friends and patients into his eighties. He kept abreast of the clinic's business, and remained involved in its operation through his physical presence and his permanent seat on the Board of Governors. And his nephew saw to it that the older man was kept fully informed and that all major decisions were carefully checked with his Uncle Doc. In the 1946–47 planning with Randy which had produced the Lovelace Foundation, Uncle Doc had at least tacitly abdicated leadership of the overall enterprise, including his clinic, in favor of Randy. But he was not hesitant afterward to contribute his views when he thought

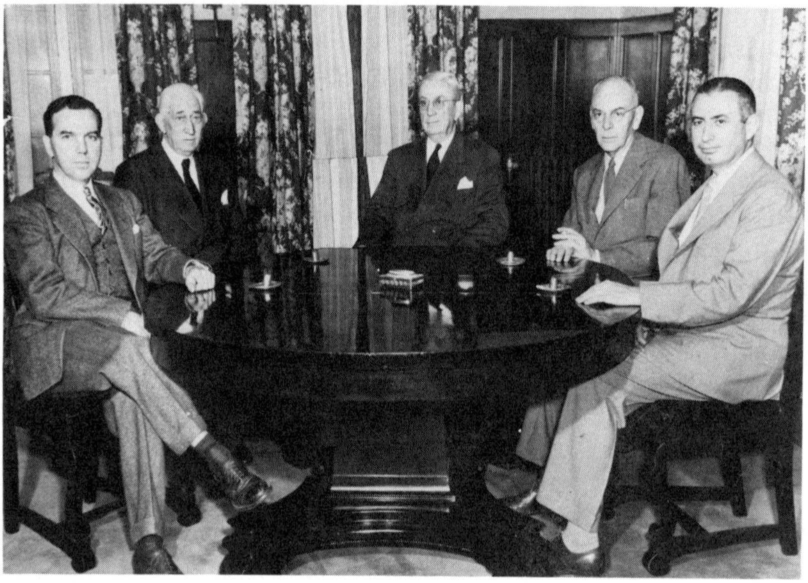

Lovelace Clinic's first Board of Governors, September, 1947. Left to right: Dr. H. L. "Jan" January; Dr. Edgar T. Lassetter; Dr. William Randolph Lovelace I; Dr. Lee Monroe Miles; and Dr. William Randolph Lovelace II.

that his experience and the wisdom of his years might bear on a problem; and his place and prestige within the organization were scrupulously protected by his nephew. They were never seen to disagree openly, although those close to them suspected that their confidential discussions were often thorough, frank, and perhaps sometimes heated. Dr. Lovelace I consistently emphasized to Randy the centrality of the clinic within the overall scheme of things in the Lovelace operation, and he took particular pains to emphasize at every opportunity the old-time ethic of taking care of the patient first and foremost. Keeping the clinic and its staff focused on the indispensability of *personalized* patient care of the highest quality possible was his raison d'être within the clinic structure during the last decades of his life—along with watching the clinic's finances. Into the 1950s, the clinic's telephone number rang at his home at night when the switchboard was closed. Physicians on the clinic's staff expected his calls late into the night: "Mrs. Ortega out in

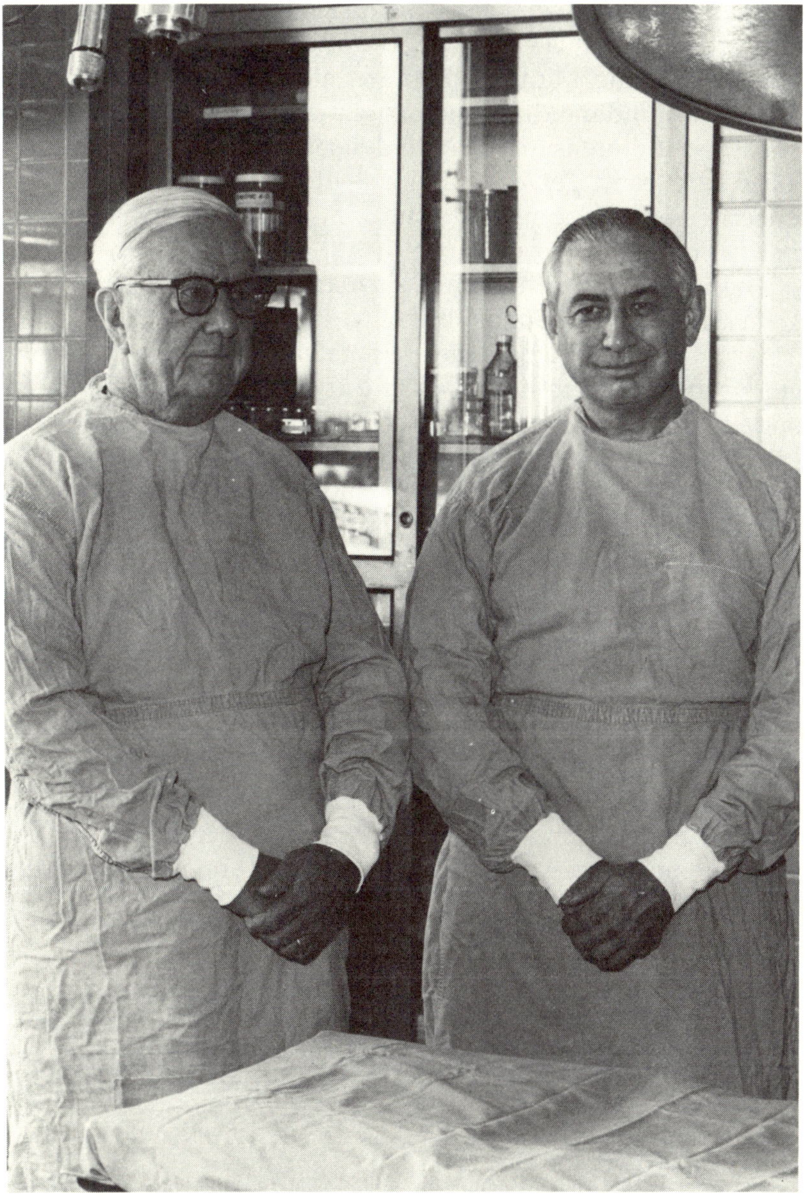

The two Drs. Lovelace in maturity, 1963.

Alameda just called with a bellyache. Do you suppose you could take care of it?"[28] It is entirely appropriate that his last recorded statement in the minutes of the clinic's Board of Governors came in a mundane discussion of clinic procedures: "Dr. Lovelace asked if there is any way to determine how many patients call in and can't get an appointment."[29] To the last, he was concerned about the patients and, not unreasonably, about the clinic's volume of patients.

The remarkable growth and increasing sophistication of the Lovelace Clinic combined with the swift development of Bataan Hospital to produce a patient-care capability of noteworthy range and strength during the fifties and sixties. As its founders intended, the Lovelace institution quickly claimed a leadership role in making top-quality health care available to a large portion of the Southwest. Probably more impressive, however, because more improbable, was the speed with which the New Mexico institution developed medical research and educational programs of sizable dimensions, which, in some cases, achieved national and international repute. That, too, was a central part of Randy Lovelace's dream; and his vision and confidence invigorated the young Lovelace Foundation as it set to work on those challenges in the late 1940s. More rapidly than even its optimistic, hard-driving director might have imagined, the Lovelace Foundation was soon disposing of multimillion dollar research budgets and playing a prominent part in one of the nation's most dramatic adventures, its manned space-flight program.

28. Several of the clinic's longtime physicians mentioned this to me. One of them, Dr. Robert Massey, remembered accidentally going back to sleep after one such late-night call, and then being awakened by the taxi that Dr. Lovelace had sent for him. Massey interview.

29. Lovelace Clinic, Board of Governors, Minutes, 27 June 1967.

FIVE

The Foundation Years

The Lovelace Foundation began its research and educational efforts in late 1947–1948 under the most primitive conditions. The doctors' offices in the crowded bank building in downtown Albuquerque provided no facilities for medical research, and no equipment was available beyond the normal instruments and appliances associated with a clinical practice employing about a dozen doctors. There were no personnel specially charged with research and/or educational responsibilities, for the Lovelace staff was constituted exclusively of hard-pressed clinicians who attended large numbers of patients daily. And the infant foundation did not start its work with large sums of working capital at its disposal. All it really had was a dream buoyed by the conviction of young Dr. Lovelace that much was possible.

In particular, he was convinced that, with luck, he might be able to parlay the federal government's increasing general interest in medical research, as well as the aviation industry's expanding demand for medical support of its enterprises, into a way to acquire the funding necessary to generate a moderately sized and aggressive research plant. Additionally, the profits of the Lovelace Clinic (and its credit) would serve to get things underway and would continue thereafter to provide one prominent element in the general support of the foundation's research and educational efforts. He could also count on the encouragement and pledges of support that he had received from the distinguished figures recruited for the foundation's Board of Trustees. Nevertheless, when the prospects of the new institution were soberly weighed, it was clear that special genius and good fortune were essential to its success.

Pivotal to that success was the first researcher Randy Lovelace hired in July 1947, just weeks before the foundation's formal incorporation. This was the brilliant physician and scientist Dr. Clayton S. "Sam" White, who remained at the center of the Lovelace Foundation's research program for almost the entirety of its first thirty years. The thirty-five-year-old White had already compiled a list of achievements that marked him as a talent of special distinction. A native of northern Colorado, he had attended the University of Colorado on an academic scholarship, and had earned a B.A. degree in psychology with grades high enough to claim Phi Beta Kappa distinction; yet he still found time and energy to win election as president of the student body and to earn all-conference honors as an end on the football team. Graduation in 1934 was followed by a year of graduate study and teaching in the university's Psychology Department; then, his college career was crowned by selection as a Rhodes scholar.[1] After three years at Oxford University, he earned an A.B. in physiology and logged a year and a half of credit in medical school. Upon his return to Colorado, he finished medical school in 1942, working in a year of full time faculty teaching and research in the process; then he spent the remainder of World War II and two postwar years in the U.S. Navy.

The navy put Sam White to work in medical research. For a time, he concentrated on respiratory physiology and problems using a low-pressure chamber at the Naval Air Station in Alameda, California; then, he completed flight-surgeon's training at the Naval School of Aviation Medicine in Pensacola, Florida, where he taught and did research until he was transferred to research duties at the navy's Flight Test Center in

1. Interestingly, Sam White's seemingly inimitable collegiate career at the University of Colorado was closely paralleled a few years after his graduation by his younger brother, Byron "Whizzer" White. Byron was also a Phi Beta Kappa and an all-conference (as well as All-American) football player, who followed undergraduate schooling with study abroad as a Rhodes scholar. Byron White went on to study law at Yale where—naturally—he led his class. He is presently an Associate Justice of the U.S. Supreme Court.

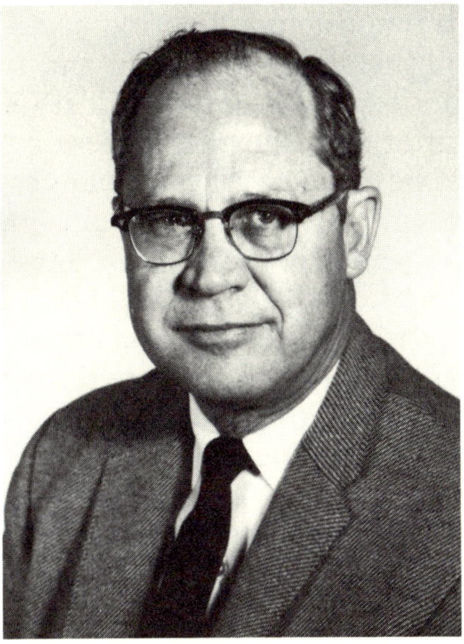

Dr. Clayton S. White, director of research of the Lovelace Foundation in a 1968 photograph.

Patuxent, Maryland. Some of his work at Pensacola and Patuxent required interaction with the air force's Aero Medical Laboratory at Wright-Patterson Air Force Base, Ohio, which was then under the command of Major Randy Lovelace. Of mutual interest to the two young physician-scientists was detailed work on oxygen masks, liquid oxygen converters, and other special equipment required in high-altitude flight. Their mutual respect and friendship was quickly sealed, and two to three years later, when Randy Lovelace began to search for staff for the new Lovelace Foundation, Sam White was high on his list. The Coloradan's quick and inquiring intellect, combined with his passion for and experience in aviation medicine, convinced Dr. Lovelace that he was a natural for the risky but promising enterprise in Albuquerque; and Sam White accepted the challenge in the summer of 1947. It was a partnership that would last beyond Randy Lovelace's death in 1965, for Sam White remained committed to the vision of a world-class medical research center that Randy had shared with him in mid-1947. He was Dr. Lovelace's successor as president of the foundation, serving as its leader during ten critical years of rapid change and adjustment. Randy Lovelace was the rare charismatic talent who possessed both the vision and daring necessary to perceive opportunity and the ability to seize it and to make things happen. He was not especially interested in (or good at) the careful development of plans for the efficient execution of an assignment, nor did he characteristically manifest the patience and perseverance essential to the successful completion of a project. Restless and inclined to move on, he often left the development and fulfillment of many of his ideas in Sam White's capable hands, and his friend's abilities (and nerves) were always more than sufficient to the task. The two men constituted an unusually effective team at the helm of the Lovelace Foundation, with one's talents complementing those of the other.[2]

When Sam White came on board in the late summer of 1947, he comprised, with Randy, the entire research staff of the new foundation. However, since there were no facilities or equipment available and no money to support research at that time, he spent much of his time in seeing clinic patients while developing his own personal contacts and research opportunities, particularly those within the aviation industry. For example, he won consulting contracts with Douglas Aircraft Corporation to study CO_2 buildup in airplane cockpits, and he shared with Randy and other staff physicians as needed the work of performing physical examinations of airline pilots from several of the major airline companies as well as test pilots from West Coast test centers like Edwards Air Force Base. With the clinic's distinguished radiologist Dr. Jack Grossman, he initiated several research projects, including work in laminography and radioisotope studies; but extensive, large-scale research at Lovelace clearly had to await appropriate quarters and funding.[3] Some progress was made in late 1949, when Dean Edward Castetter of the University of New Mexico's Graduate School loaned the Lovelace Foundation an old temporary navy building on the university campus. In using foundation money to

2. On the working relationship, mutual respect, and friendship between the two men, see particularly the series of interviews with Dr. White. Dr. Clayton S. White, interview with the author, Albuquerque, 14 October 1985 and passim.

3. Ibid.

purchase basic equipment, White fashioned a small respiratory physiology laboratory in the building; hired a full-time biochemist to help in it; and began work to establish 17-keto steroid standards for clinical and research purposes, while developing the basic techniques fundamental to operating a laboratory in respiratory physiology. Several clinicians—including rheumatologist Dr. Clarence "Bud" Kemper, thoracic surgeon Dr. Rodger MacQuigg, and orthopedist Dr. Lew Overton, as well as Dr. Grossman—got their own individual research projects going in the limited time available away from their busy practices; but the small scale of Lovelace Foundation research work was reflected in the modest 13,317 dollars spent during the startup period ending in 1949. All of that modest sum (except for the Douglas contract revenues) had come from contributions to the foundation and funds accruing to it from the clinic's operations.[4]

The opening of the new Lovelace Clinic Building on Gibson Boulevard in late 1950 afforded new prospects for the foundation, and its research effort quickened perceptibly. The new structure included more than four thousand square feet of space for research operations, and by the end of the next year no fewer than nine different contract projects, most funded by the U.S. Air Force, and a similar number of clinical projects were under investigation in the new facility.[5] The institution was obviously still in flux, feeling its way tentatively while exploring various funding options and research possibilities. Nevertheless, the *Annual Research Report* for 1950–1951 indicated clearly the predispositions of the foundation's leadership. While acknowledging the possibilities of shaping the foundation's research program to serve local needs—for example, the state of New Mexico had no toxicology laboratory, and the region's

4. Lovelace Foundation for Medical Education and Research, Board of Trustees, Minutes, 15 January 1950; White interview.

5. Lovelace Foundation for Medical Education and Research, *Annual Research Report,* 1950–51, pp. 1–4. The annual reports of the foundation were comprehensive documents compiled and written every year by Dr. White in his capacity as Director of Research. Including up to three hundred pages of statistics, charts, graphs, narrative, and analysis, these reports are vitally important source materials for the history of the Lovelace institution.

cattle and mining industries needed medical-research support—the report identified aviation medicine as the clear central focus of the organization's work to that point:

> Certain nationally important industries, of which air transportation and airplane design and manufacture are two excellent examples, very much need a medical organization with a strong research potential to which they may turn for help in many fields.[6]

Underscoring the Albuquerque research center's increasing slant toward aviation medicine was the national and even international prominence it achieved in 1951 through its role in the organization and administration of a high-powered medical symposium on the physics and medicine of the upper atmosphere. Randy Lovelace promoted the idea for such a gathering, and won official support for the undertaking through his contacts and his position on the Scientific Advisory Board of the U.S. Air Force. Once he had engineered the selection of the new Albuquerque research foundation as the agent for running the symposium, a large-scale organizational challenge to the still small foundation's staff was set in motion. The purpose of the meeting was to pull together the available data, other information, and expertise essential to planning future research related to manned flight toward the top of the earth's atmosphere. In November 1951, a galaxy of national and international scientists—astrophysicists, aeronautical engineers, biologists, radiobiologists, toxicologists, and aviation medicine specialists, among others—assembled at the U.S. Air Force School of Aviation Medicine in San Antonio for the mutual sharing of information and views. The conference "put the Lovelace Foundation on the map as a research center for aviation medicine,"[7] and the visibility and prestige achieved via the symposium consti-

6. Ibid.

7. Clayton S. White, "The Lovelace Years," in J. A. Loeppky and M. L. Riedesel, eds., *Oxygen Transport to Human Tissues: A Symposium in Honor of Dr. U.C. Luft* (New York and Amsterdam: Elsevier Biomedical, 1983), p. 7; White interview. The proceedings of the symposium were published under the auspices of the Lovelace Foundation as *Physics and Medicine of the Upper Atmosphere: A Study of the Aeropause,* ed. Sam White and Otis O. Benson (Albuquerque, New Mexico: University of New Mexico Press, 1952).

tuted a vitally needed boost for the fledgling research center, helping it to establish contacts and associations that would prove to be of use to it in later years.

Lovelace's budding reputation and its special expertise in aviation medicine were fortified in late 1950 by the addition to the staff of Dr. Walter Boothby, recently retired from a distinguished career at the Mayo Clinic. Dr. Boothby, one of the authentic pioneers in aviation medicine who had been Randy Lovelace's mentor at Mayo (see pp. 53–56), accepted his former student's invitation to come to Albuquerque in 1950. It was hoped that the dry, desert climate of the Southwest might help the veteran researcher's asthma, and Randy Lovelace was eager to pay a debt of gratitude to the physician-scientist who had done so much to advance his own career. Dr. Boothby spent only a little more than two years in Albuquerque, but the luster of his name further enhanced the growing reputation of the Lovelace Medical Center among those interested in aviation or aerospace medicine.

Dr. Boothby's was the most celebrated name on the Lovelace staff prior to his death in 1953, but at the very beginning of the following year, a physiologist of worldwide repute, Dr. Ulrich C. Luft, joined his fortunes with those of the new research center. This distinguished scientist had built a brilliant record as a young physician-scientist in his native Germany during the 1930s, focusing his imaginative studies in respiratory physiology. Dr. Luft had been clever enough to combine his interest in the impact of high altitudes on respiratory physiology with Himalayan mountaineering in some of the most famous climbing expeditions of the 1930s.[8] By the 1950s he was especially well known and highly regarded for his research on hypoxia and high-altitude acclimatization, much of which had been carried out during his tenure as chief of Aviation Physiology at Berlin's Aeromedical Research Institute from 1942 to 1945. From wartorn Germany he emigrated in 1947 to the U.S. Air Force School of Aviation Medicine in San Antonio, and a

8. For information on Dr. Luft's life and career, see his file in the Lovelace Medical Center archives and the symposium volume dedicated to him (see n. 7, above). See also Dr. Ulrich C. Luft, interview with the author, Albuquerque, 11 October 1985 and passim.

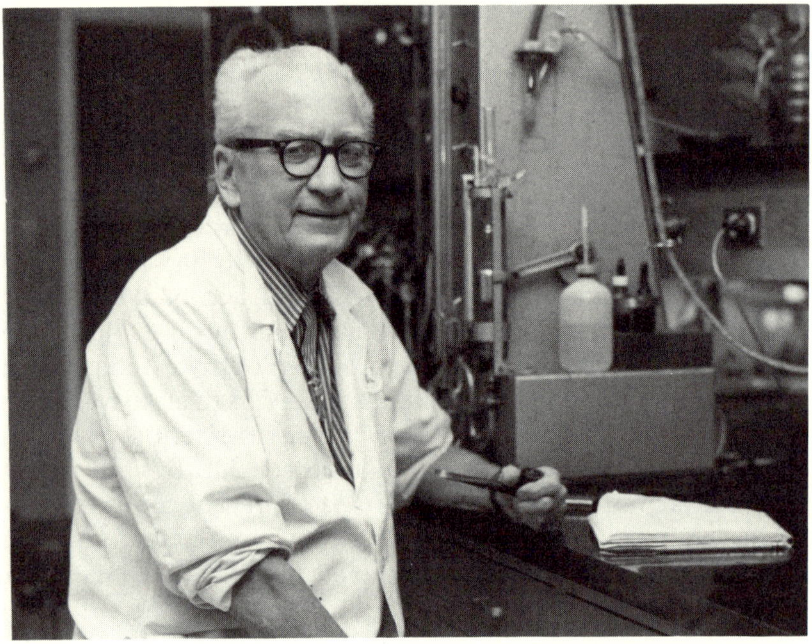

Dr. Ulrich C. Luft, head of the Lovelace Foundation's Physiology Department from 1954 until his retirement in 1980.

little over six years later he gave in to Randy Lovelace's entreaties and agreed to join the Lovelace Foundation in Albuquerque as head of its Physiology Department. From 1954 until his retirement in 1980, he was the best known and one of the most prolific scientists on the Lovelace staff. His list of scholarly publications stretches chronologically from a 1936 study of hypoxemia in a major German scientific journal to articles and reports produced in the 1980s, and his contributions to his field have made him one of its major figures during this century. His presence in Albuquerque was generally acknowledged as one of the primary elements in the building and consolidation of the Lovelace institution's reputation as a center of excellence in aviation medicine.[9]

9. Dr. Donald E. Kilgore, interview with the author, Albuquerque, 18 November 1984 and passim.

Although the early focus of the Lovelace Foundation was on aviation medicine—an emphasis manifest throughout the 1950s and evident from the numerous U.S. Air Force research contracts, grants, consultancies, and additional contracts with private firms in the aviation construction and airline industries, as well as in the selection of the Albuquerque center to do the basic medical screening for the Project Mercury astronauts (see pp. 132–138)—it was an Atomic Energy Commission contract, initiated in 1951, which first made significant sums of money available to the Lovelace researchers; and in the process, it greatly stimulated growth of the foundation's staff and facilities. This blast and shock biology program was a contractual effort sponsored until 1960 by the AEC's Division of Biology and Medicine and continued thereafter with support of the Defense Atomic Support Agency. Throughout the 1950s it was by far the foundation's largest research effort, and ultimately its longest lived, stretching out over thirty-five years. Born in the aftermath of the Hiroshima and Nagasaki atomic blasts, it was part of the initial scientific investigation of those phenomena. Several major research centers in this country and elsewhere set to work in trying to understand the effects of nuclear explosions, but most of the early studies concentrated on ionizing radiation and thermal effects, with relatively little attention directed to the biological consequences of the blast and shock aspects of high-yield explosions. The program set up at Lovelace in 1951 was aimed toward understanding the biological effects of rapid variations of environmental pressure induced by explosions, the damage produced by energized debris, and the consequences of accelerative and decelerative whole-body displacement.[10]

Sam White, the architect of this first major contract effort of the Lovelace Foundation, thought that the AEC work was "a special opportunity for a fledgling foundation trying, with the help of the Clinic, to set up basic medical and educational programs"; and he insisted on the scientific overlap between the study areas central to the blast and shock biology program

10. White, "The Lovelace Years," p. 7.

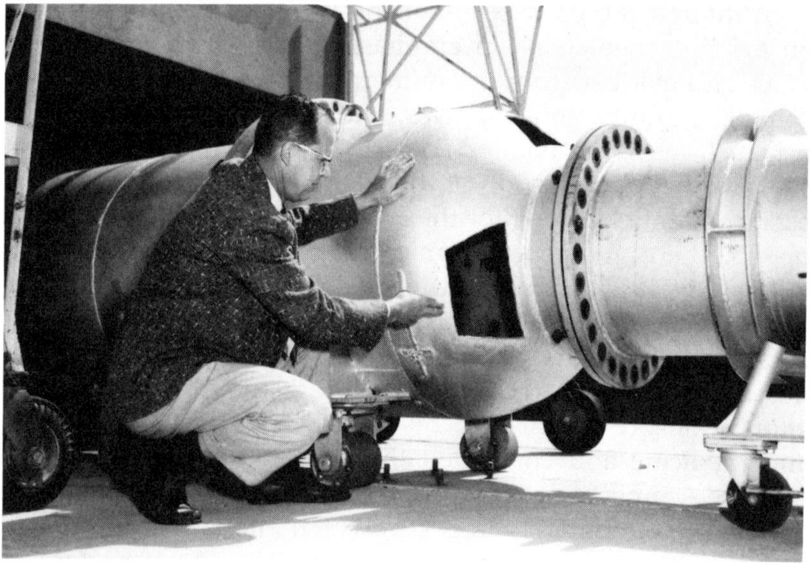

Dr. Sam White, in a 1958 photograph, inspects one of the shock tubes designed and fabricated by Lovelace researchers as part of the Lovelace Foundation's blast and shock biology program.

and those already under preliminary development at the Albuquerque institution. Beginning with an initial contract of 25,000 dollars in 1951, the blast and shock biology program (in later years called the biodynamics program) ultimately stretched over more than thirty years, providing nearly 4 million dollars to the foundation budget and producing more than ninety scientific publications during its first fifteen years alone.[11] The funds available through this contract helped enormously in the development of the foundation's staff (see pp. 125–126) and in the buildup of an inventory of sophisticated equipment at the Lovelace plant and even more sophisticated scientific and administrative expertise.

Most of the work was concentrated at a field site located in a secure area on Sandia Base approximately nine miles from

11. See Lovelace Foundation for Medical Education and Research, *Annual Research Report*, for yearly summaries of the progress of the blast and shock biology program. Those reports are detailed through 1971–1972, while later volumes offer a summary.

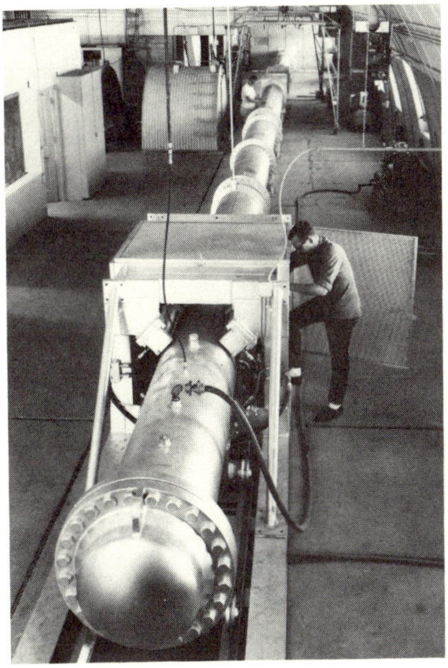

The shock tubes employed by Lovelace researchers in their blast and shock biology program were used to simulate the shock waves associated with nuclear explosions.

foundation headquarters on Gibson Boulevard, where a number of unpretentious buildings—including an old hangar, a Navy Quonset hut, two or three Butler buildings, animal barns, and kennels—made up the government-owned facility. (Eight departments housed in headquarters on Gibson contributed to the program's investigations.) On numerous occasions, however, the research team involved in this project worked at distant sites, including three different and extended visits to the AEC's Nevada test site (in 1953, 1955, and 1957) as well as to other test locales in California, Alberta, Canada, and Australia. As the first major project conducted by the Lovelace Foundation, the blast and shock biology program afforded the organization's planners and administrators vitally needed experience in the logistics, management, and financing of large-scale research efforts; and the program's strongly interdisciplinary nature was important in shaping the basic ethos and patterns of work and cooperation within the new research center. This first AEC contract, for example, was fundamentally the responsibility of the foundation's Departments of Comparative Environmental Biology, Engineering, Pathology, and Physics; but it

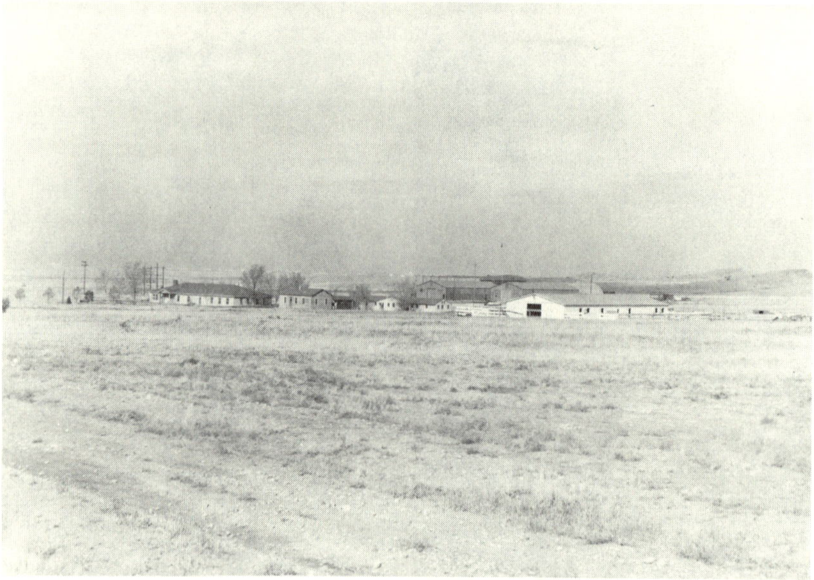

The field site on Albuquerque's Sandia Base used for Lovelace's blast and shock biology program. This 1953 photograph emphasizes the isolation of the site.

also involved the Departments of Biomathematics and Computer Systems, Medical Illustration, Veterinary Medicine, and the Library in support roles. This Lovelace work received much favorable attention from the nation's scientific community and had immediate impact in the fields of civil defense planning, nuclear safety engineering, and elsewhere. It was a strong start for the Lovelace research team and commands a place of high honor in the institution's history.

A second AEC contract, initiated in 1961, eventually dwarfed the blast and shock biology program, at least in size and visibility. A broad spectrum environmental research effort, originally called the fission inhalation program, was initiated by a contract with the AEC dated 1 June 1960. At the invitation of the AEC's Division of Biology and Medicine, the same agency with which Lovelace had worked during the start of the blast and shock biology program, the Lovelace Foundation undertook development of a program to help evaluate the potential

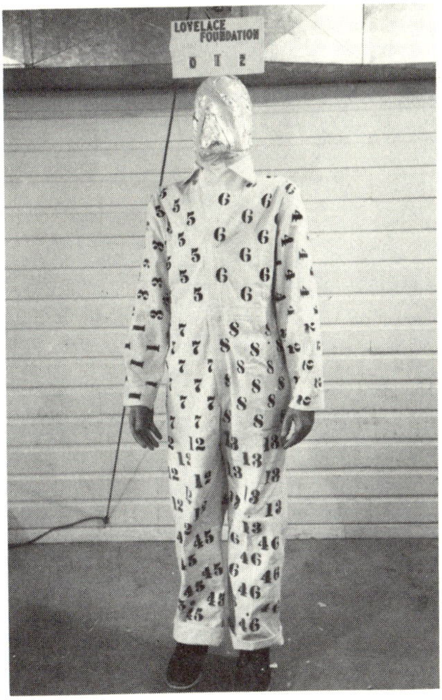

An anthropomorphic dummy used to simulate human targets during the Priscilla and Smoky shots at the Nevada test grounds in 1957. Lovelace researchers participated in the 1953, 1955, and 1957 nuclear test series as part of their blast and shock biology work.

short-, intermediate-, and long-term hazards of the release of fission products, both radioactive and inert elements, into the environment. The program's overall objectives were to use experimental animals in studying the biological consequences of inhaling soluble and insoluble fission products, singly and as mixtures, so that various levels of exposure could be related to biological effects. Swiftly, the new program came to dominate the foundation's research effort. As early as its third full year, fiscal year 1962–63, the fission product inhalation program claimed 743,000 dollars of the foundation's research budget, an impressive 45 percent of the total; and by the time of Randy Lovelace's death two years later, its expenditures had risen to 1.9 million dollars, or about 55 percent of the total.[12] By the 1960s, the two AEC-originated programs commanded up to three-quarters of the Lovelace Foundation's total research budget

12. Since the fission product inhalation program came to full maturity only in the 1970s and 1980s, its development is sketched more fully in the next chapter.

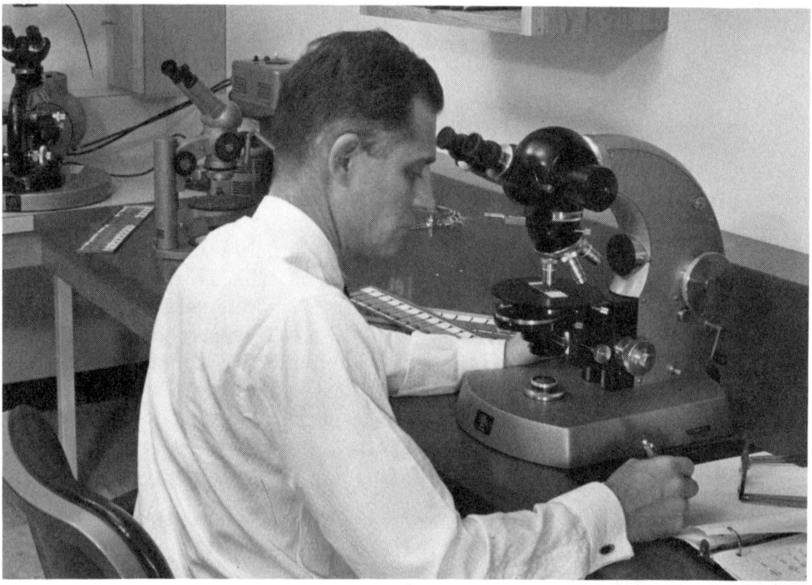

Pathologist Dr. Tom Chiffelle joined the Lovelace staff in 1951 and participated centrally in its research programs while heading the Clinic's pathology department. He gave more than 35 years of distinguished service to the institution.

and a commensurate level of its manpower and institutional attention.

During those early years, however, other contractual efforts played important roles in the foundation's early research program. Particularly interesting was a National Institutes of Health-funded program on physiologic and psychologic aging, which extended throughout the decade of the sixties. Initiated in 1960 by a contract with the Federal Aviation Agency and then taken over by the NIH, this investigation involved studies of pilots using a battery of physiological, psychological, and clinical tests. It aimed at evaluating the levels of normal function in American males as they varied with time and age; and by project's end in 1969, test data had been compiled on a sample group of 457 pilots. This program, which came to the Albuquerque foundation through the efforts of Randy Lovelace and Dr. A. H. Schwichtenberg, head of the foundation's Department of Aviation Medicine, was one of Lovelace's million-dollar programs that depended basically on the foundation's experience with test pilots and its special focus on aviation medicine. Other important contractual efforts of the 1950s and early 1960s included a NASA-sponsored space medicine information analysis program, which focused on collection and analysis of information from all disciplines, biological as well as physical, relating to the biomedical aspects of operating manned spacecraft;[13] a Defense Atomic Support Agency-sponsored combined injury program that studied hazards associated with exposure to all significant combinations of environmental variation produced by nuclear explosions; and an AEC program on selected aspects of weapons effects, a million-dollar contract which was a spinoff from the blast and shock biology work. By the mid-1960s, contract research constituted from 80 to 90 percent of the overall research program of the Lovelace Foundation, with most of it occurring in the sphere of what might be called environmental studies; and the Albuquerque center had established a strong and growing reputation for reliability and excellence within the several areas of its special expertise.

Basic-science research at the new foundation developed more slowly than the environmental programs, all of which were supported by extramural money. Dr. Luft's Physiology Department, which emphasized basic scientific study (as opposed to clinical or environmental), was always able to attract outside support for its work; and the Department of Biochemistry, headed since 1952 by Dr. Bernard B. Longwell, and the Department of Microbiology, chaired also since 1952 by Dr. W. Everett Clapper, built commendable records in basic-science studies despite carrying heavy service laboratory responsibilities for the clinic. Drs. Longwell and Clapper were veteran teacher-researchers whom Sam White had "liberated" from the University of Colorado Medical School when the foundation began its basic de-

13. One of the fruits of this project was the publication of a compendium of information on aerospace medicine which has become a standard reference work of the field: Emannuel M. Roth, ed., *Compendium of Human Responses to the Aerospace Environment*, 4 vols. (Albuquerque, N.M.: Lovelace Foundation for Medical Education and Research for NASA, 1968).

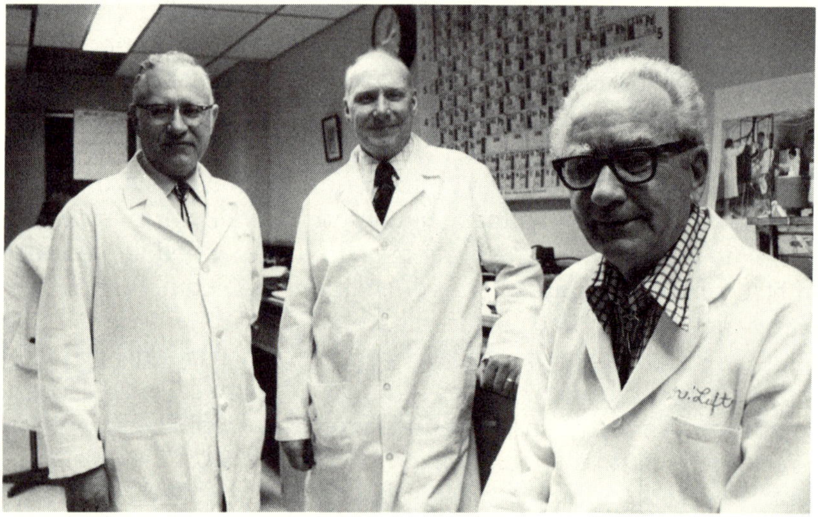

Three of the Lovelace Foundation's veteran researchers (left to right): hematologist Dr. Bruce Wimer, who served the Clinic and Foundation from 1962 to 1981; Dr. Eugene Rypka, microbiologist for the Clinic and Foundation from 1971 to the present; and Dr. Luft.

partmental expansion in the early 1950s.[14] Other foundation departments—physics, hematology, pathology, and radiology prominent among them—were active to a somewhat lesser degree in basic-science research, with their efforts limited by personnel and financial constraints. Although the Lovelace Foundation had quickly built a broad departmental structure for its work—there were twenty-one departments by 1965—they were all thinly staffed. Only those departments, such as aerosol physics or comparative environmental biology, which were fed by extramural contract money, had anything resem-

14. The tradition of excellence established in the Microbiology Department was especially strong. After Dr. Clapper's retirement, the department was headed by Dr. Eugene Rypka, whose work using automation and clustering techniques to identify microflora was started in support of the fission product program, but went on independently to attract worldwide attention. Dr. Rypka's contributions to automating clinical and research microbiology laboratories, developing effective approaches to handling large data bases, and to the emerging field of artificial intelligence have brought much favorable attention to the foundation.

bling adequate staffs; and it is within that context that the foundation's contributions to basic scientific research must be viewed. On balance, it was a good record, and that was the judgment of Dr. White, the foundation's director of research, in 1961: "To date the basic research output is fairly creditable, even though departments are not yet developed in sufficient depth to realize the full power of mutual cooperation and work between as well as within the several disciplines."[15]

Clinical research at the Lovelace Foundation developed most slowly of all. This was not from lack of interest, for members of the Lovelace Clinic staff, in particular, were engaged in clinical studies from the very beginning. However, those practicing physicians had to subordinate their research interests to their clinical responsibilities, with the result that research often suffered. Dr. Jack Grossman managed to sandwich a number of clinical research projects, including imaginative cancer therapy work, within his already full clinical workload. Dr. Roy Goddard, a clinic pediatrician and part-time employee of the foundation, conducted a number of studies focused on development of new infant resuscitation equipment and techniques. Clinic orthopedist Dr. Lew Overton (assisted by Dr. Grossman) did extensive anatomical studies of the cervical spine, with special attention to related clinical observations. Rheumatologist Dr. "Bud" Kemper conducted extensive studies of therapeutic agents which were of potential use in treatment of arthritis as well as in other arthritis research. Most of these early clinical research projects were relatively small-scale ones, and many of them were dependent entirely or partially on intramural funding. So long as the foundation's budget for research remained limited and clinicians felt constrained to focus their schedules on patient care, clinical research at the Lovelace Foundation was bound to develop slowly.

Only in the early 1960s did clinical research within the Albuquerque center begin to move forward strongly. Increasing numbers of clinic staffers—39 physicians in 1965—dedicated a

15. Lovelace Foundation for Medical Education and Research, *Annual Research Report*, 1959–1960, p. 162.

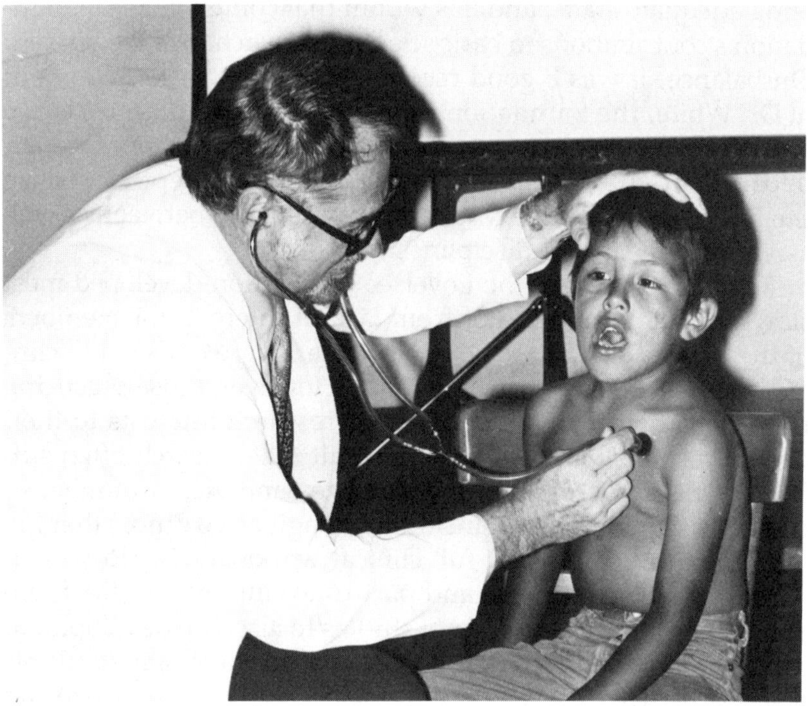

Dr. Roy Goddard, pediatrician at the Lovelace Clinic from 1952 to 1974 and head of the Lovelace Foundation's extensive pediatric research efforts, is shown here examining a patient at a Taos Indian Health Clinic.

portion, at least, of their time, without extra compensation, to clinical research projects. (Five other physicians and two PhDs were employed jointly by the foundation and clinic.)[16] A number of those projects, which were usually studies of a limited and well-defined scope, attracted outside financial support, and almost all of the foundation's clinical research work was assisted by general research support grants available through the NIH. But only one clinical effort was of sufficient size to command a place among the foundation's major research efforts; this was a cardiovascular research program initiated in 1958,

16. Lovelace Foundation for Medical Education and Research, *Annual Research Report*, 1964–1965, pp. 127–30. Again, for details on the development and thrust of clinical research at the Albuquerque institution, see the individual yearly reports.

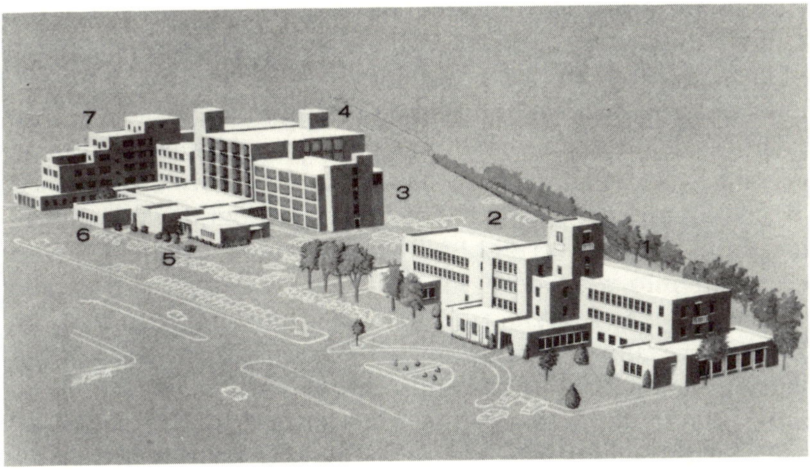

Lovelace Clinic, Lovelace Foundation and Bataan Hospital in 1965. (1) Original Clinic Building and (2) Baird Memorial Wing; (3) Lassetter Laboratory Building; (4) Lovelace Foundation Building (later named the William R. Lovelace I Building); (5) Radiation Therapy Building; (6) Obstetrics and Gynecology Building; and (7) Bataan Memorial Methodist Hospital.

with intramural funds and personnel largely supplied by the Lovelace Clinic, but supported from 1962 forward by a NIH grant. By 1965 the cardiovascular research program, which concentrated on the development and application of equipment and apparatus for cardiac surgery and cardiopulmonary resuscitation—especially the use of deep hypothermia in cardiovascular surgery and new techniques for heart-lung resuscitation—had produced nearly two dozen scientific papers, two prize-winning educational and training movies, and a large number of training sessions covering heart-lung resuscitation and research conducted before local, state, and national groups. It was a solid clinical investigation, bringing much credit to the Lovelace institution; and it indicated the range and caliber of work possible, despite the distance of the Albuquerque researchers from the national citadels of clinical research. Adequate financial support was the key, and money was a chronic limitation to the expansion of clinical research at Lovelace during this period.

Key to the dynamic development of the foundation's research program in the fifties and sixties was the rapid provision of extensive new research facilities. Within fourteen years, the solitary, borrowed quonset hut on the UNM campus—Sam White's first respiratory physiology lab—gave way to an impressive complex of eight modern buildings on the Gibson Boulevard headquarters site plus others on two field sites. Beginning with no room at all, the Lovelace Foundation by 1963 owned 330,000 square feet of space. The building program, which produced this almost overnight transformation of tough east mesa scrubland into a modern medical complex unrivaled in the Southwest, was both daring and yet difficult because of its speed. For example, provision had to be made not only for the creation of the laboratories and other working space essential to the foundation's booming research program, but also for the needs of its tenant, the Lovelace Clinic, which rented office space, examination and treatment rooms, laboratory facilities, and other necessities from the foundation. Since the clinic staff more than tripled during that period, the demand placed on the foundation is apparent.

In the building boom of the late 1950s and early 1960s, the guidance and tangible assistance of the foundation's Board of Trustees was crucial. As one illustration, the board consistently followed a policy of overbuilding—striving to be "space long"—throughout the era of rapid growth. If a building with two stories and a basement and including 25,000 square feet was immediately needed, the unvarying policy of the board was to authorize construction of a facility with *four* stories and the basement, with the upper two floors roughed in in shell fashion for later completion and use. It was both a financially prudent approach and a policy whose inherent flexibility accommodated the dynamism of the foundation and clinic in a remarkable way. And the board members backed up their wisdom and advice with their money. The role of the foundation's trustees and other friends in the construction of the Lovelace Clinic Building, the first structure on the Gibson Boulevard campus, has already been described (see pp. 83–87). In each of the subsequent building projects, the largesse of the Lovelace Foundation trustees was conspicuous. Through his family foundation, David Baird gave 350,000 dollars; and Albert Mitchell added another 100,000 dollars for construction in 1952 of the Baird-Mitchell laboratory addition to the original Clinic Building. John Jay

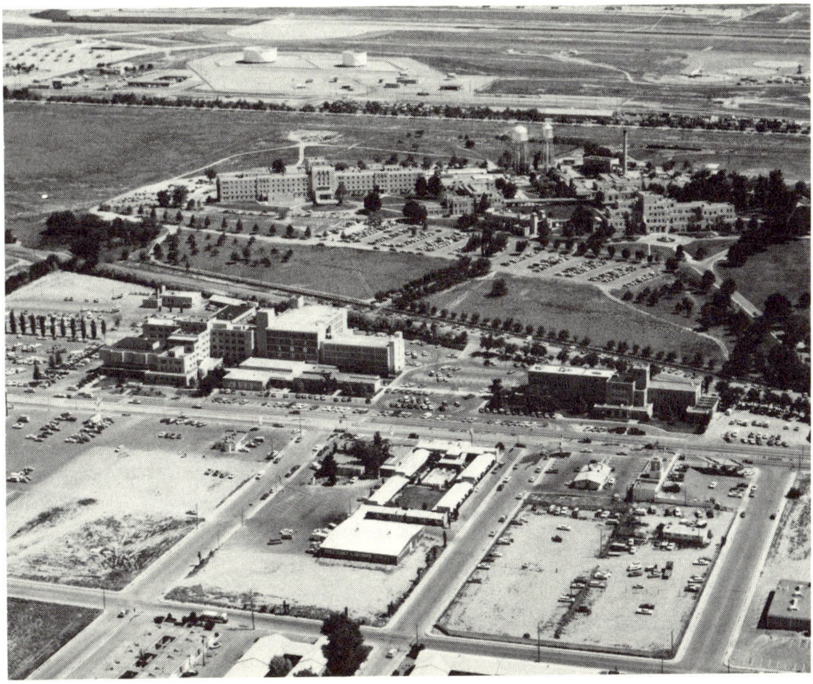

Aerial shot of the Lovelace facilities in the late sixties.

Hopkins, Floyd Odlum, and others financed the construction in 1953 of the Radiation Therapy Center; and another trustee, Ellis Hall, contributed the 85,000 dollars necessary to equip it with the purchase of a Cobalt-60 Rotational Teletherapy Unit, the second of its kind in the country. When the William R. Lovelace Building (originally called simply the New Lovelace Foundation Building) was constructed at a total cost of 2.6 million dollars in 1963, trustees and other friends of the foundation produced 560,000 dollars of the total funding.[17] The stunning

17. To illustrate the financing of such a large building project, the 2.6 million dollars for the W. R. Lovelace Building was produced through the following means:

$560,000	private donations
$230,000	Hill-Burton (federal government) grant
$466,000	U.S. Public Health Service grant
$1,336,000	mortgage
$2,592,000	

Lovelace Foundation for Medical Education and Research, *Annual Research Report*, 1962–1963, p. 158.

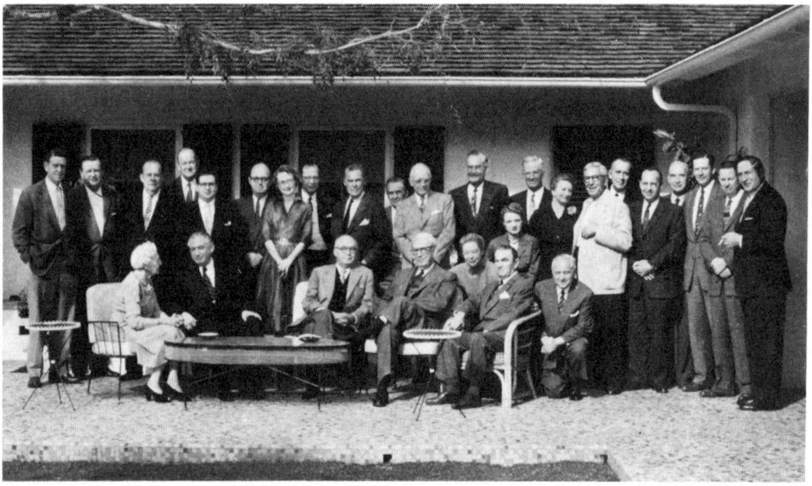

The Lovelace Foundation Board of Trustees (with several foundation administrators and friends) at its 1950 annual meeting, held at John Hertz's Canoga Park, California estate.

physical growth of the Lovelace enterprise could hardly have been accomplished without the faith and support of its farsighted and generous board.

All of the various statistical measurements available reflect the remarkable development of the Lovelace Foundation during the years between its birth in 1947 and the climacteric of Randy Lovelace's death in 1965. For example, Table 2 shows the budgetary growth of the foundation's program up to 1965. By that year the Lovelace researchers had spent more than 13.6 million dollars on its research and educational work, 83 percent of which had come from external sources via contracts, grants in aid, consultancies, and other miscellaneous sources. Until fiscal year 1961, intramural sources—primarily the rent paid by the clinic to the foundation—had supported approximately one-third of the cost of the research and educational program; but with the phenomenal growth of the foundation's contract research, especially the fission products inhalation work, that percentage slipped markedly even though total revenues from clinic rent as well as donations continued to rise. The giant

Table 2 Lovelace Foundation Program Costs and Income, 1947–1965

Fiscal Year	*Total Expenditures*	*Extramural Income**	*Intramural Income#*	*(% of total)*
1947–49				
1950	$13,000			
1951	$51,000			
1952	$159,000	$136,000	$23,000	(14%)
1953	$214,000	$180,000	$34,000	(16%)
1954	$328,000	$190,000	$139,000	(42%)
1955	$414,000	$236,000	$179,000	(43%)
1956	$397,000	$216,000	$181,000	(46%)
1957	$416,000	$283,000	$134,000	(32%)
1958	$481,000	$298,000	$183,000	(38%)
1959	$614,000	$396,000	$218,000	(36%)
1960	$737,000	$480,000	$258,000	(35%)
1961	$928,000	$727,000	$201,000	(22%)
1962	$1,305,000	$1,141,000	$163,000	(13%)
1963	$1,642,000	$1,474,000	$168,000	(10%)
1964	$2,504,000	$2,259,000	$245,000	(10%)
1965	$3,445,000	$3,263,000	$182,000	(5%)

*Contracts, Grants-in-aid, and Miscellaneous Sources.
#Rent and Donations.
Source: Lovelace Foundation for Medical Education and Research, *Annual Reports.*

expansion in total money spent was paralleled by equally large staff increases during this time of growth. (See Table 3.) By 1965 the 326 staff members of the Lovelace Foundation—with two-thirds of them full-time foundation employees and the rest shared between the foundation and clinic—commanded an annual salary payroll of 1.6 million dollars.[18] They also constituted one of the most impressive pools of scientific and other professional talent in the region, many of whom possessed skills available nowhere else. By 1965 the foundation had accumu-

18. The physicians of the Lovelace Clinic were members of a professional association which contracted with the foundation, and thus their salaries are *not* included in the 1.6 million dollars, nor are those of other employees of the clinic. All of these figures are compiled from the annual reports of the foundation.

Table 3 Lovelace Foundation Staff, 1950–1965

Fiscal	*Full Time*		*Part Time*		*Unpaid**		*Total*		*STAFF*
Year	*Prof.*	*Tech.*	*Prof.*	*Tech.*	*Prof.*	*Tech.*	*Prof.*	*Tech.*	*TOTAL*
1950	1		2	2			3	2	5
1951	4	4	5	2			9	6	15
1952	6	13	8	2	1		15	15	30
1953	10	15	9	6	1		20	21	41
1954	16	15	8	2	2		26	17	43
1955	17	14	8	3	4	2	29	19	48
1956	17	10	8	7	5	2	30	19	49
1957	18	13	8	8	5	2	31	23	54
1958	22	13	9	7	7	4	38	24	62
1959	24	18	10	8	7	4	41	30	71
1960	24	19	8	8	23	5	55	32	87
1961	36	34	11	8	31	3	78	45	123
1962	47	61	9	13	33	6	89	80	169
1963	52	105	9	17	33	4	94	126	220
1964	59	152	8	21	44	4	111	177	288
1965	60	177	14	27	44	4	118	208	326

*Clinic employees working on foundation projects.

Source: Lovelace Foundation for Medical Education and Research, *Annual Reports.*

lated more than 2.3 million dollars in scientific equipment, and its library—15,400 scientific books and bound serials—was the largest of its type in the region. When Director of Research White gathered his statistics at the end of every fiscal year to make his annual report on the foundation's progress, the numbers expressing the institution's performance grew steadily larger and the graphs accompanying them continued their sharp movements upward.

Medical education was one of the cardinal interests of the Lovelace Foundation's creators when they started the enterprise in 1947, for there were few educational programs of any description available anywhere in the Southwest. But, medical education programs developed very slowly in the foundation's early years, essentially because the founders and first managers of the foundation quickly realized the impossibility of doing everything at once. Money was the basic problem; while research programs might be initiated and nourished with the assistance of outside funding, there was little money available to assist educational programs. Consequently, the Lovelace planners decided to emphasize their research program while determining to "catch up" later on the educational work.

As early as 1948, nine Lovelace Clinic staff members were participating as "faculty" or attending physicians in the two new internal medicine and general surgery residency programs, which were begun that year at the VA Hospital adjacent to the clinic property. Throughout the early fifties, Lovelace physicians—Dr. White in particular—did some graduate teaching in physiology in association with the University of New Mexico. However, independent and more elaborate teaching programs had to await both sufficient funding and the formal approval of Bataan Hospital as a teaching hospital capable of supporting such things as residency programs. When that particular technical hurdle was passed in 1954, cautious planning for a modest educational effort began. Working in tandem with the Lovelace Clinic and Bataan Hospital, the Lovelace Foundation made formal application in 1954 for approval of residencies in internal medicine, radiology, and pathology, and simultaneously began an extern program aimed at junior- and senior-year medical students interested in serving three-month clerkships in the clinic and at Bataan Hospital. Shortly thereafter, the first formal education committees were formed in both the clinic and the foundation, and in 1956 all of the preliminary study and work came to fruition in an in-house educational program involving eight externs and the first three residents (in medicine and pathology) on site.[19] The direct costs of the foundation's education program stood at a modest 7,137 dollars that year, though indirect costs swelled the total considerably.

A clinic hematologist, Dr. Samuel Painter, served on a part-time basis as the foundation's first acting director of education, doing the essential work that launched the extern program and

19. The application for residencies in general surgery and radiology were denied for technical reasons, primarily the insufficient number of free beds available for teaching purposes at Bataan Hospital and the inadequate patient-case volume to support them.

the first residencies. At the beginning of 1958, Dr. Painter was succeeded by a distinguished medical educator, Dr. Burgess Gordon, former president of the famous Woman's Medical College in Philadelphia. Dr. Gordon arrived in Albuquerque with great expectations and commensurate energies, but his tenure at Lovelace was relatively brief and not entirely happy. In his first *Annual Education Report,* written in early 1958 after little more than two months on the job, Dr. Gordon sketched plans for the rapid expansion (at significantly greater costs) of the foundation's educational program. He anticipated a rapid growth in the residency programs through the enlargement of the two existing programs and the addition of several others; a continuation and increased emphasis of the extern program; the full-scale participation by Lovelace in the new nursing education program just beginning at UNM in 1958; a medical-technician program to be conducted in association with the VA Hospital, UNM, and the Bernalillo County Indian Hospital, which was also slated to begin in 1958;[20] as well as seminars, guest lectures, and other educational programs intended for practicing physicians and other health professionals in the area—which today would be called continuing education programs.

Most of these proposals were already the subject of some discussion on the Lovelace campus when Dr. Gordon arrived, and two or three were already in place or in advanced planning stages. What *was* different was Dr. Gordon's intention to move quickly from the discussion and planning stages to action within each of these educational spheres as well as others; and clearly his efforts would cost much more than the educational program was accustomed to spending. (In fiscal year 1956–57, for instance, the foundation's total educational costs were just under 15,000 dollars.) Few on the Lovelace campus opposed Dr. Gordon's ambitious program on philosophical grounds, but many questioned the practicality of pushing forward so quickly and

20. For some years, the clinic's head of radiology, Dr. Jack Grossman, had been directing his own two-year X-ray technician program, and by 1958 seven of his pupils had passed the certification exams given by the American Registry of X-ray Technicians. Lovelace Foundation for Medical Education and Research, *Annual Education Report,* 1956–1957, p. 5.

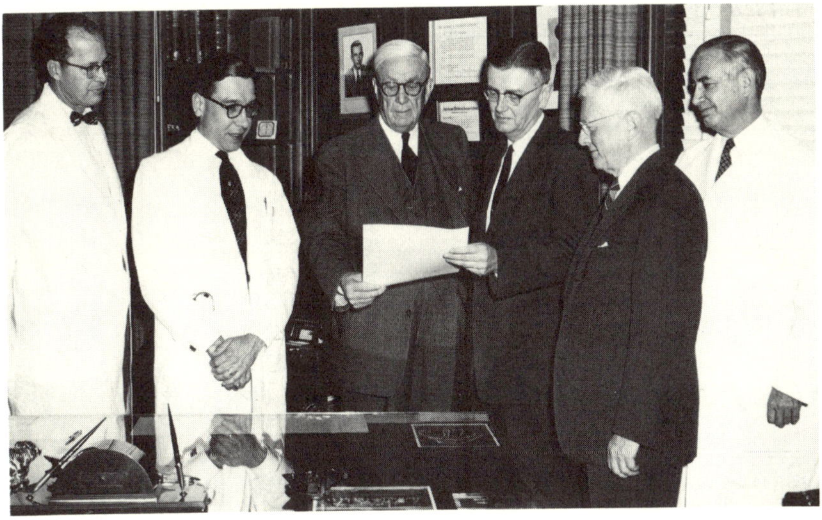

Clinic-Foundation leaders with a visiting lecturer from the Mayo Clinic, Dr. Karl J. Olsen. Left to right: Dr. Sam White; Dr. Robert Massey; Dr. W. R. Lovelace I; Dr. Olsen; Dr. Burgess Gordon; and Dr. Randy Lovelace.

broadly (and expensively). Table 4 shows clearly the dimensions of the new director of education's achievements—a tripling of the budget for education in his first year on the job and maintenance thereafter of the higher sum—but it also provides a certain clue to his relatively quick departure in 1960. The foundation could not yet afford the kind of educational program that Dr. Gordon proposed, and he left Albuquerque in 1960 for a position at the American Medical Association headquarters.

To the perennial concern about the cost of extensive educational efforts, a new element was added at the end of the 1950s. As part of an increasing national concern about a possible doctor shortage, serious discussions began in New Mexico regarding the possibility of establishing a medical school in the state.[21] Consequently, an element of uncertainty began to enter

21. For details on the background discussions and planning of the medical school at the University of New Mexico, see Jake W. Spidle, Jr., *Doctors of Medicine in New Mexico: A History of Health and Medical Practice, 1886–1986* (Albuquerque, N.M.: University of New Mexico Press, 1986), pp. 309–18.

Table 4 Lovelace Foundation Educational Program Costs, 1956–1965

Fiscal Year	*Direct Costs**
1956	$7,137
1957	$14,796
1958	$45,073
1959	$47,244
1960	$43,907
1961	$28,073
1962	$38,052
1963	$28,473
1964	$16,844
1965	$24,355

*Does not include any portion of the physician–educators' salaries, overhead, or other incidental costs.

Source: Lovelace Foundation for Medical Education and Research, *Annual Reports.*

into Lovelace's educational planning. From its first, tentative educational efforts of the fifties, the Lovelace administration had sought to coordinate its limited programs with those of the University of New Mexico. Those efforts had been only marginally successful, and there was considerable feeling within the Lovelace institution that the university authorities, for whatever reasons, were not fully committed to cooperating with them.[22] Disappointment at the university's unenthusiastic attitude contributed to the serious discussion on the Lovelace campus of the possibility of the foundation forming its own medical school. In retrospect, such an idea seems wildly ambitious, given the enormous sums required by medical schools of the 1970s and 1980s, but the idea was not considered to be farfetched in the context of the late 1950s. Many of the basic elements of a medical school were already in place or in process

22. As early as 1955, Director of Research White complained in his annual report. "All efforts to establish liaison with a degree-granting institution on a formal basis have failed. The University of New Mexico has not acted favorably, though informal contacts continue to be useful." Lovelace Foundation for Medical Education and Research, *Annual Research Report,* 1954–1955, p. 38. Private comments on the subject were undoubtedly more pungent.

of development by the Lovelace institutions, and given sufficient money and commitment, progression toward rounding out their programs would be relatively easy. In his 1958–59 annual report on the operations of the Lovelace Foundation, Dr. White discussed the proposition:

> Last, it is felt wise to call attention to a local trend that is not directly connected with the Foundation and not yet given much thought; namely, the increasing tempo of activities in Albuquerque aimed at establishing a medical school at the University of New Mexico under State support. Though the time scale is not yet clear and no final decisions have been made, one can say that within two to five years a 2-year medical program might well be underway, followed in five to ten years by a full 4-year curriculum.
>
> Such a development, if approved and implemented, cannot help but be a factor of significance in the future developments of the Foundation and therefore is also a matter deserving the close attention of the Director and the Board of Trustees. Currently, the Foundation is the only organized group in the Southwest that is active in medical education and research. One might go farther and argue that the Foundation should undertake the organization and operation of a small medical school with very high standards, along with a related hospital. Certainly, such a course is well within the objectives set forth in the Foundation's charter, fits well with the staff that has been assembled, and presents a challenge well worth very serious consideration.[23]

At its February 1960 annual meeting, the foundation's Board of Trustees passed a resolution "that the Lovelace Foundation could, without commitment, make a broad study in regard to the establishment of a medical school."[24] Lovelace quickly abandoned its interest in creating its own medical school, largely

23. Lovelace Foundation for Medical Education and Research, *Annual Research Report*, 1958–59, p. 47.

24. Lovelace Foundation for Medical Education and Research, Board of Trustees, Annual Meeting, Minutes, 28 February 1960.

because of the rapidly developing momentum gained by advocates of a state-supported school at the University of New Mexico. Instead, the Lovelace physicians and scientists—Randy Lovelace and Bob Massey, in particular—enlisted themselves and the weight of their institution in doing the political work and planning necessary to make the idea of a state school a reality. The Lovelace contribution to the success of that effort—the UNM School of Medicine opened in 1964—was substantial and a source of pride to those involved. However, the emergence of the idea of a "Lovelace Medical School" was particularly interesting as an indication of the conceptual scale of thought by the foundation's leaders and as a sign of the frustration felt by the Lovelace staff—at least some members—in their efforts to cooperate with the local university.

By the time of Randy Lovelace's death in 1965, the educational mission of the Lovelace Foundation was solidly launched. At that time, its program included five approved residency programs (in medicine, surgery, radiology, pathology, and aerospace medicine) with spaces approved for up to twenty-five residents;[25] an externship program for medical students which, in 1964–65, brought seventeen medical students to the Lovelace-Bataan facilities from such schools as the University of Oklahoma School of Medicine, Philadelphia's Jefferson Medical College, the University of Colorado School of Medicine, the Louisiana State University School of Medicine, and the University of California, Los Angeles, School of Medicine; a postgraduate fellowship program, focused mainly on the foundation's Physiology Department; a School of X-ray Technology approved by the AMA's Council on Medical Education; an active visiting-professor program; and miscellaneous other educational projects. It was a solid start for an effort that had begun essentially only a decade earlier.

No account of Lovelace history would be complete without at least passing reference to one of the most dramatic episodes

25. In fiscal year 1964–65, the foundation, with the assistance of Bataan Hospital, supported eight residents.

in the institution's long history. In late 1958, the Lovelace Foundation was asked to accept responsibility for medical selection of the first group of American astronauts, the seven men who would fly in Project Mercury. Within six months, the assignment had been completed with skill and dispatch, and the name of the relatively unknown Southwest foundation and clinic was featured in prominent national journals such as the *New York Times* and *Life* magazine. A measure of national visibility and even prestige was achieved by the Albuquerque medical center through its astronaut screening program, and the effort remains a proud chapter in the institution's corporate memory.

Since the late 1940s, the Lovelace Foundation and Clinic had been extensively involved in both the clinical examination of airline and aviation-industry test pilots and in aviation medicine research. It was this experience and acknowledged expertise which make the Lovelace center a natural site for the medical screening of the astronauts. When NASA was created in October 1958, the center was already at work on development of a test protocol for the clinical examination of space pilots. Funded by a U.S. Air Force grant, the Lovelace Foundation began work on this problem in early 1958. Responsibility for the project had been assigned to a recent addition to the Lovelace staff, a newly retired air force physician-scientist, Brigadier General Albert H. Schwichtenberg. Dr. Schwichtenberg, an ophthamologist by training, had served a distinguished career in the air force, including six years as command surgeon of the Air Defense Command in Colorado Springs immediately prior to his retirement in the spring of 1958. During his service years, he had become good friends with Randy Lovelace; and upon retirement he accepted the latter's long-standing invitation to come to Albuquerque to join the foundation as head of its Department of Aviation Medicine and Bioastronautics.[26] Dr. Schwichtenberg was a key addition to the Lovelace staff; his long familiarity with the structure and operations of the military and his extensive network of contacts, combined with his first-rate man-

26. Dr. A. H. Schwichtenberg, interview with the author, Albuquerque, 20 February 1985.

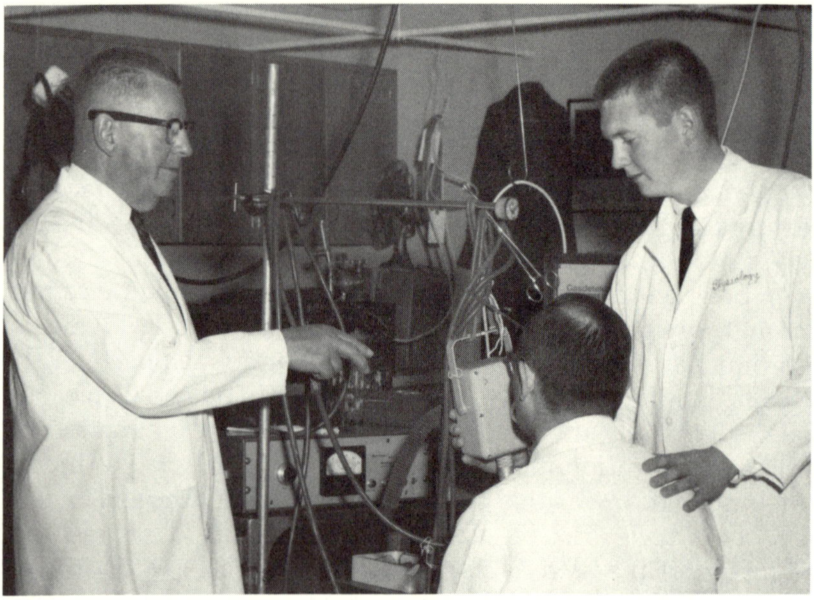

Dr. A. H. Schwichtenberg, head of the Foundation's Aviation Medicine department from 1958 to 1970, at left, and medical student William Rutherford, right, inspect test apparatus in this photograph.

agerial abilities and his devotion to aviation medicine, uniquely prepared him for the assignments that he undertook at Lovelace from 1958 to 1970.[27]

In early February 1959, the first of six groups of astronaut aspirants, a total of thirty-two men, began the clinical examination process in Albuquerque.[28] The full test regimen required a total of seven and one-half days and three evenings (see Table 5) and involved six basic components: a medical and aviation history; a physical examination; laboratory tests; a radiographic

27 Dr. Schwichtenberg, a soft-spoken and compassionate man, is crudely burlesqued in the 1983 movie based on Tom Wolfe's *The Right Stuff* (New York: Farrar, Straus, Giroux, 1979), where he is presented as the epitome of a cold and insensitive bureaucrat. He, in particular, and the Lovelace Clinic, in general, are also presented quite unsympathetically in the Wolfe book; see pp. 88–95.

28. For Randy Lovelace's charming personal description of the examination process, see his article "Duckings, Probings, Checks That Proved Fliers' Fitness," in the 20 April 1959 issue of *Life* magazine.

Table 5 Schedule for the Lovelace Astronaut Screening Program

	SUNDAY
On arrival	Complete Cornell Medical History Forms and IBM Forms.
	Collect first stool specimen Sunday night or Monday morning.
12:00 midnight	Nothing to eat, drink or smoke after midnight until after completion of laboratory tests on Monday morning.
	MONDAY
	Nothing to eat, drink or smoke on arising.
	Collect first stool specimen Monday morning if not collected Sunday night; turn in stool specimen to Laboratory Control Desk.
8:00 a.m.	Report to Laboratory Control Desk on first floor of Lassetter Laboratory Building for tests listed below:
	Complete Blood Count; Sedimentation Rate
	Special Hematology Smear; Cholesterol
	Blood Sugar; Blood Grouping
	Non-Protein Nitrogen; Rh Factor
	Serology; Urinalysis
9:00 a.m.	Report to flight surgeon, third floor of Clinic Building, for general history and physical examination.
10:30 a.m.	Report to receptionist for referral for ECG; also, obtain instructions for preparation for proctoscopic examination Monday afternoon.
12:00 noon	Lunch
1:30 p.m.	Report to Clinic Emergency Room for proctoscopic examination.
2:00 p.m.	Report to receptionist for referral for dental and sinus x-rays.
3:00 p.m.	Report to receptionist for referral for vector-cardiograms.
Evening	No restrictions on eating, drinking or smoking.
12:00 midnight	Nothing to eat, drink or smoke after midnight.
	TUESDAY
	Nothing to eat, drink or smoke on arising.
	Collect second stool specimen Tuesday morning if not collected Monday night.
	Turn in stool specimen at Laboratory Control Desk.
	Collect entire urine specimen for radiation physicist.
7:00 a.m.	Report to radiation physicist in Radiation Therapy Building for total body water determination. Turn in urine specimen to him.
11:00 a.m.	Report to Laboratory Control Desk for BSP liver function test.
12:00 noon	Start 24-hour urine collection.
	Lunch
1:30 p.m.	Report to Cardiology, first floor of Clinic Building, for tilt-table tests.
3:00 p.m.	Report to receptionist for referral for lumbar-spine x-rays.
4:30 p.m.	Report to receptionist for instructions for preparation for gastric analysis and the colon x-rays on Wednesday morning.
Evening	No restrictions on eating or drinking. Do not smoke after 7:00 p.m. until after blood volume determination Wednesday afternoon.
12:00 midnight	Nothing to eat, drink or smoke after midnight.

Table 5 continued on page 136.

Table 5 continued

	WEDNESDAY
	Nothing to eat, drink or smoke on arising. Do not smoke until after completion of blood volume determination, Wednesday afternoon.
8:00 a.m.	Report to Laboratory for gastric analysis.
9:30 a.m.	Immediately following gastric analysis, report to X-ray Department for colon x-rays.
12:00 noon	Turn in 24-hour urine collection at laboratory control desk.
	Lunch
1:30 p.m.	Report to Physiology Department, first floor of Clinic building, for blood volume determination.
2:30 p.m.	Report to Ophthalmology Department, second floor of Clinic building, for ophthalmological examination.
Evening	No restrictions on eating, drinking or smoking this evening.
12:00 midnight	Nothing to eat, drink or smoke after midnight, until after completion of stomach x-rays on Thursday morning.
	THURSDAY
	Nothing to eat, drink or smoke on arising.
8:00 a.m.	Report to receptionist for referral for stomach, chest and esophagus x-rays.
	Upon completion of x-rays, you may eat breakfast if time permits.
10:00 a.m.	Report to Carco Air Service for flight to Los Alamos.
11:00 a.m.	Total body counter—K^{40} determination.
3:30 p.m.	Report to Physiology Department, first floor of Clinic building, for pulmonary function testing.
	No restrictions on eating, drinking or smoking this evening.
	Wash hair before going to bed; do not re-apply oil, spray, or anything on hair until after completion of electroencephalograms on Friday afternoon.
	FRIDAY
	You may eat a light breakfast.
8:00 a.m.	Report to Physiology Department, first floor of the Clinic building, for hydrostatic weighing.
8:30 a.m.	Report to Physiology Department for exercise tests.
9:30 a.m.	Report to receptionist for referral for audiograms.
10:30 a.m.	Report to Physical Medicine Department, second floor of Clinic building, for neurological examination.
12:00 noon	Lunch
1:30 p.m.	Report to receptionist for referral for electroencephalograms.
4:00 p.m.	Report to Otolaryngology Department, third floor of Clinic building, for ENT examination.
Evening	No restrictions on eating, drinking or smoking this evening.
	SATURDAY
	You may eat breakfast.
9:00 a.m.	Report to flight surgeon, third floor of Clinic building.

Source: Lovelace et al., "Selection and Maintenance Program for Astronauts," pp. 683–84.

examination; physical competence and ventilatory efficiency tests; and a final evaluation.[29] Thanks largely to the thorough planning and preparation by Dr. Schwichtenberg and his colleagues as well as the full cooperation of the Lovelace staff, the entire operation was completed successfully and according to plan. The Lovelace physicians and scientists involved in the process uniformly remember it with pride and satisfaction, for it was a smooth professional job from start to finish.[30] However, it was not a pleasant experience for the astronaut candidates. There were, for example, blood counts and sperm counts, barium enemas, electrical stimulations, and tubes to be swallowed for gastric analysis. The examination involved poking, jabbing, prodding, and so many ways of measuring that successful candidate John Glenn later observed, "I didn't know the human body had so many openings to explore."[31] Their attitude toward their Lovelace visit was also colored by the natural antagonism toward doctors existing among pilots. As Deke Slayton, another successful candidate, insisted years later, "You must remember that the doctors have the power to sit you down!"[32]

Prior to their arrival in Albuquerque, the astronaut candidates were instructed not to talk about the purpose of their visit, and the Lovelace authorities made every effort to avoid unwanted public attention to the operation. (The local newspapers did not carry news of the story until after the examinations were over.) Nevertheless, throughout the period of preparation for the exams, the exams themselves, and the weeks and months thereafter, there was a special electricity in the

29. For full details of the testing process, see W. Randolph Lovelace II, A. H. Schwichtenberg, Ulrich C. Luft, and Robert R. Secrest, "Selection and Maintenance Program for Astronauts for the National Aeronautics and Space Administration," *Aerospace Medicine* 33 (1962):667–84. See also Mae Mills Link, *Space Medicine in Project Mercury* (Washington, D.C.: National Aeronautics and Space Administration, 1965), esp. pp. 48–53.

30. See, for example, Dr. D. Angus McKinnon, interview with the author, Albuquerque, 25 October 1984; Dr. Ulrich C. Luft, interview with the author, Albuquerque, 11 October 1985; Kilgore interview; and Schwichtenberg interview.

31. Cited in Lovelace, "Duckings, Probings, Checks," p. 117.

32. Donald K. "Deke" Slayton, interview with the author, Houston, Tex., 12 May 1986. However, Slayton went on to suggest that the hopeful astronauts did respect the work of the Lovelace physicians—even if they tilted in the direction of "over-thoroughness"—and developed a particular affection for "Dr. Randy."

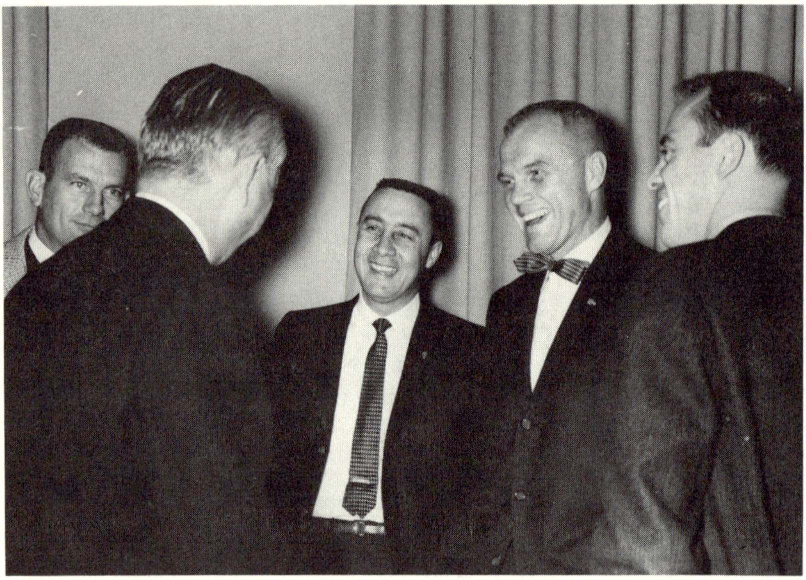

In this 1960 photograph, Dr. Randy Lovelace (back to the camera) shares a joke with four of the Project Mercury astronauts. Left to right: Donald K. "Deke" Slayton; Virgil "Gus" Grissom; John Glenn; and Alan Shephard.

center, especially when references to the Lovelace Clinic began to appear in the national press. The astronaut testing program had climaxed the quick emergence of the distant Albuquerque medical center to the first rank in the field of aviation and aerospace medicine.

No further testing was done at Lovelace, for NASA recognized the need to develop its own independent medical capability because of the scale of its operations and the centrality of medical issues within its manned space program. However, the Lovelace Foundation and Clinic remained in close contact with the space program, carrying out extensive contract work for the agency and consulting with it on a regular and intimate basis. Most concretely of all, the Lovelace center remained closely connected to NASA through its leader, Randy Lovelace. After the astronaut testing program, Randy accepted ever greater responsibilities within the NASA effort. He was chairman of its Special Advisory Committee on Life Sciences from 1959 to 1963; senior consultant to its Office of Manned Flight in 1963-

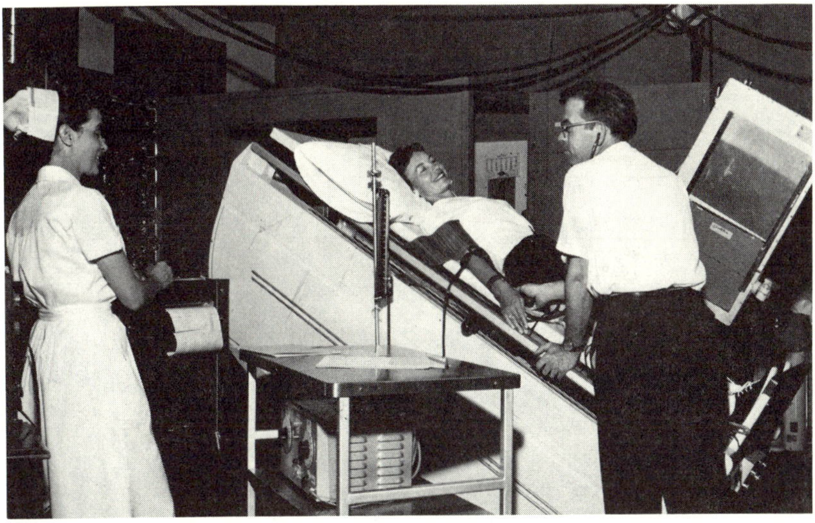

After the successful experience with the Project Mercury astronaut candidates, the Lovelace Foundation tested a group of women pilots to establish their suitability for space flight. In this 1962 photograph, Dr. Robert Secrest, right, tests one candidate on a tilt table. Longtime Lovelace nurse Sadie Rhoades, left, assists.

64; and finally, became its director of space medicine in April 1964, a post he held until his death a year and a half later.

On a bright, crisp Sunday afternoon, 12 December 1965, Randy and Mary Lovelace, with their charter pilot, Milton Brown, boarded a twin-engine Beechcraft Travelair in Aspen, Colorado, for the pleasant two-hour flight home to Albuquerque. They had spent the morning in the resort town checking on the progress of the condominium they were building and visiting with Dr. Alvin Eurich and his wife. (Dr. Eurich was president of the Aspen Institute for Humanistic Studies and a member of the Lovelace Foundation's Board of Trustees.) Within a half hour or so, their plane was down, the casualty of a navigational error that took it into a blind mountain canyon too narrow to allow a 180 degree turn.[33] All three passengers were killed,

33. Details of the tragedy and the search for the lost plane may be found in Elliott, " 'On a Comet, Always.' ", pp. 351–53 and 380–83; the Luft interview; and in the Ulrich C. Luft and W. Randolph Lovelace II files in the Lovelace Medical Center archives.

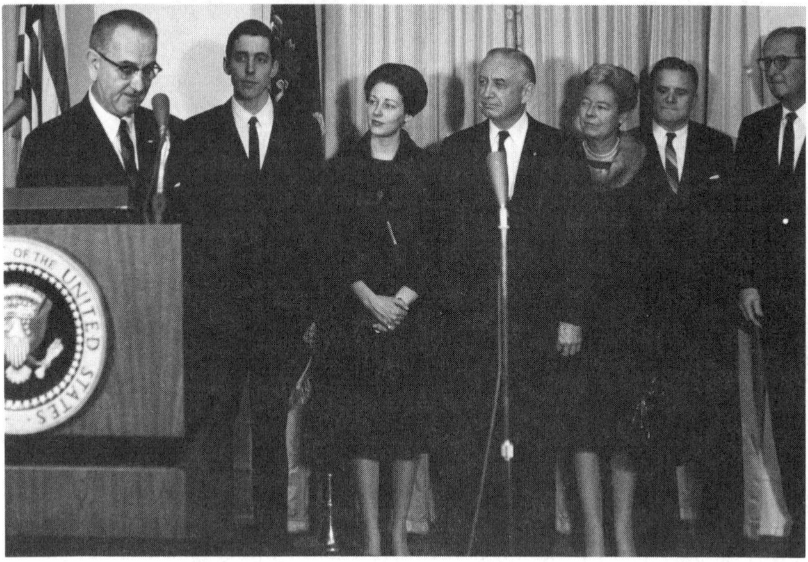

The swearing-in ceremony in which Dr. Randy Lovelace became Director of Space Medicine for NASA, 21 April 1964. Left to right: President Lyndon B. Johnson; Dr. John and Christine Sellman (son-in-law and daughter of Randy and Mary Lovelace); Dr. and Mrs. Lovelace; James Webb, NASA Administrator; and Senator Clinton P. Anderson, senior senator from New Mexico and old friend of the Lovelace family.

Randy apparently instantaneously. The wreckage of the plane was first spotted on Tuesday, December 14, but it was not until Wednesday that searchers could push through the heavy snow to the crash site to begin the sad work of bringing the bodies out. Ironically, that December 15 was the day of the rendezvous deep in space of Gemini 6 and Gemini 7, a day of triumph within the American space program Randy Lovelace had done so much to advance.[34]

34. President Lyndon Johnson noted the irony in an official statement:
"A day of great achievement in space was marred by news of the death of Dr. William R. Lovelace II. His life was too short, although his legacy to space medicine will endure and will be a source of assurance to future astronauts whose names and deeds are yet unknown."
Statement by the President on the Death of the Chief Medical Adviser to NASA. December 16, 1965.

ALBUQUERQUE JOURNAL Tuesday Morning, December 14, 1965

Dr. Lovelace, Wife Missing

Albuquerque Doctor On Aircraft Overdue From Colorado Town

ALBUQUERQUE JOURNAL Wednesday Morning, December 15, 1965

Clouds, Snow Mar Search for Lovelaces

ALBUQUERQUE JOURNAL Thursday Morning, December 16, 1965

All on Lovelace Plane Are Found Dead

Newspaper headlines told a tragic story.

The institution that Randy Lovelace had done so much to create and shape was shaken to its core by, first, the news of the overdue plane, and then by the even more fearful tidings which followed. Randy Lovelace was a rare man, one who would be grievously missed both personally and as the inspiring, driving mainspring of one of the Southwest's premier medical institutions. His loss was felt with special keenness by his eighty-two-year-old Uncle Doc, who was already in declining health and never recovered from the loss of his nephew, passing away in December of 1968. With the deaths of the founders, the Lovelace Foundation and Clinic came to the end of one momentous phase of their history and, with little specific preparation, entered another.

SIX

A New Era

DURING THE 1970s AND 1980s, the highly personalized institution fashioned by Uncle Doc and Randy Lovelace experienced perhaps more changes of sweeping dimensions than at any other period in its history. Within all three of the basic spheres of its activity—health-care delivery, medical research, and medical education—the Lovelace Medical Center experimented and adjusted to its rapidly evolving environment, yet it still managed to remain remarkably true to the traditions and principles that had shaped its birth and growth. The Lovelace Clinic went through a difficult period of redefinition in the early and mid-seventies, but it proved to be flexible and imaginative in transforming itself to meet the changed circumstances of the late twentieth-century medical marketplace. In the pioneering spirit of Uncle Doc and Randy, it charted new courses in establishing the earliest and largest health maintenance organization (HMO) in the Southwest, and it expanded its services beyond the Gibson Boulevard campus to a string of successful satellite clinics. Meanwhile, the Lovelace Foundation built its sophisticated research program into a 25-million-dollar annual enterprise that included a world-renowned toxicology-research institute and a number of clinical-research programs of broad range and creativity. The special focus on space medicine fostered in the foundation's early years slipped from center stage, but moved forward anew in the 1980s. And within the educational sphere of its charter responsibilities, the Lovelace Foundation devoted ever larger sums of money to an increasingly varied array of medical-education programs and established a major place for itself within the region's medical education system. In a time of considerable stress and challenge, the leadership of the Lovelace center picked its way skillfully through the difficult and even threatening environment and positioned the institution to face the challenges of the new century, creating a record of which its people could be proud.

In the first days of 1966, three weeks after the airplane crash that claimed Randy Lovelace's life, his Uncle Doc appeared for the first time in over two years at a regularly scheduled meeting of the clinic's Board of Governors:

> Dr. Lovelace opened the meeting stating he was happy to be with the members of the Board of Governors, but did not expect to find himself back under the current circumstances. On the other hand, he was happy that he was able to be available to assist in any way possible.[1]

His presence was an important assertion of continuity, an affirmation that things would go forward in the clinic that the eighty-two-year-old doctor had founded forty years earlier. But it was the clinic's fifty-two-year-old radiologist, Dr. Jack Grossman, who reluctantly assumed the burden of clinic leadership during the period of adjustment after Randy's death.

Dr. Grossman was a member of the "Class of 1941," which had been so important in the clinic's growth and development throughout the fifties and sixties. The quiet and scholarly radiologist did not seek leadership of the clinic, nor had he been groomed as a potential successor to Randy; but he was a twenty-five-year veteran of the institution, knew its operations and personnel, and commanded the respect and loyalty of his peers. For more than four years he shouldered the responsibility of guiding the clinic, apparently without ever developing a taste for the job or deriving much satisfaction from it. His major contribution to the institution—aside from the not inconsiderable service of holding the medical group together during the

1. Lovelace Clinic, Board of Governors, Minutes, 5 January 1966.

first years of adjustment—lay in his efforts to improve financial management within the clinic and to establish sounder fiscal and business practices. Randy Lovelace had been casual, almost cavalier, about the finances of the clinic, confident that he could square whatever financial circles presented themselves. He insisted frequently that money ought not play any role in determining good medical practice.[2] Dr. Grossman was far more attentive to the financial details of the operation, an attitude that contributed enormously to the institution's greater fiscal integrity. When Dr. Grossman took over, the clinic was operating with a deficit and had accumulated a significant debt, but by "watching the pennies" and installing tighter financial controls, the new chairman succeeded in producing a small profit within a relatively short time.

A moderate degree of democratization in the clinic's governance also marked Dr. Grossman's tenure as chairman of its board of governors. For example, the clinic's virtually all-powerful Board of Governors was a self-perpetuating oligarchy until the end of the 1960s, with its members serving eight-year terms and electing their own successors. As late as 1966 the board defended this system, arguing bluntly that

> the method of selection of the Board of Governors and its officers should provide for distinct continuity to result in sound business management. Such selection should be free of the risk of election by popular vote.[3]

However, increasing pressure from the staff physicians forced a retreat from this policy, with the board first agreeing to choose among nominees selected by staff vote, and then, in the early seventies, accepting the principle that the staff should elect

2. Interviews with clinic veterans uniformly stressed this point. One clinic colleague, who respected and admired Randy Lovelace enormously, went so far as to suggest that "it may have been a good thing that Randy died when he did"—thus indicating that there were numerous, and serious, systemic problems within the Lovelace institution that were begging for attention in the mid-sixties. Managerial reform and greatly improved financial supervision were two of the more prominent problems and required fundamental reform rather than the "fire-fighting" or "band-aid" approach which some suggested was Randy Lovelace's approach. Private communications.

3. Lovelace Clinic, Board of Governors, Minutes, 15 November 1966.

directly the governors of the board. This reform was accompanied by increased staff participation in salary determinations through an open and petitionable salary committee, an innovation of the late sixties, and the establishment of clearer and more consistent salary guidelines. In 1966 and 1967, the staff also claimed for itself a prominent role in the development of specific policies regarding the rights and obligations of clinic physicians in distributing their time among research, education, and clinical practice, a touchy subject which had generated much controversy within the institution.

Another measure of internal reform accomplished during the Grossman tenure as chairman of the clinic's board dealt with one of the most disputed and hotly criticized policies of the Lovelace institution: the restrictive covenant clause included in all of the clinic's physician contracts. By the terms of this clause, a physician who chose to leave Lovelace was barred from practicing anywhere in Bernalillo County for a period of three years without special permission of the clinic authorities. This legal restriction existed in clinic contracts as early as the thirties, and probably originated in the senior Dr. Lovelace's "betrayal" by his cousin, Dr. Loren Elliott, in the 1920s. (See pp. 36–37.) To a considerable degree, the clause made good business sense. Its supporters argued that the clinic could not be expected to bring a new doctor to town; provide him with clientele; support him while he built his practice; and then watch with equanimity while he moved downtown, taking his patients with him. In the thirties and forties, such legal and contractual restrictions were not uncommon among professional associations such as the Lovelace Clinic; and even today, they remain in use in certain circumstances. However, for many physicians, both within the clinic and outside it, the restrictive covenant clause was a highly offensive, "yellow-dog contract,"[4] a demeaning, artificial, and unethical constraint on their personal and professional freedom.

4. This is the phrase of one of the clinic's "refugees," that is, a Lovelace physician who left the place when he grew dissatisfied with it, but was forced to leave the county for three years before he could even think of practicing in Albuquerque.

Occasionally, the clause was challenged in the courts, most prominently in the mid-sixties when a clinic dermatologist, Dr. John C. Murphy, instituted legal action. When the case was decided against Dr. Murphy and the decision was upheld all the way through the New Mexico Supreme Court, the dermatologist set up his practice by simply moving across the county line to Corrales, a rural suburb of Albuquerque. (After the three-year term elapsed, he moved back into Albuquerque.) Years before, among many other clinic "refugees," Dr. Robert C. Derbyshire left the clinic to move to Artesia, New Mexico (then later to Santa Fe); Dr. Stuart Adler went to Santa Fe (then back to Albuquerque); Dr. Lou Levin moved to Belen (then returned to Albuquerque); Dr. John Parker went to Farmington; and Dr. Richard Streeper moved to Santa Fe. Some Lovelace veterans have argued, mostly with tongue in cheek, that the clinic contributed greatly to the improvement of the caliber of the state's medical practice via its restrictive covenant clause.[5] However, in the period after Randy Lovelace's death the clause came under increasing criticism within the clinic itself—its effect upon recruiting was a special concern as was the public and professional relations damage associated with it—and in early 1970 the Board of Governors finally voted to eliminate it from all contracts.[6]

The controversy surrounding the "yellow-dog contract" was largely contained within the Lovelace staff and the medical profession at large; but unfortunately, another major episode of the Grossman years came under public scrutiny. This was the rendering by a New Mexico court of the largest malpractice judgment (to that time) in the history of New Mexico medicine; the unhappy target of that judgment was the Lovelace Clinic. The essential facts of the case were never disputed. In late 1958 a three-and-one-half-year-old boy, Lawrence Lucas, was treated at the clinic for ringworm of the scalp. When the case failed to yield to conventional therapy, X-ray treatment was employed,

5. As one illustration, see Dr. Donald E. Kilgore, Jr., interview with the author, Albuquerque, 18 November 1985 and passim.

6. Lovelace Clinic, Board of Governors, Minutes, 24 March 1970.

and in the process the boy accidentally received eight to ten times the intended radiation.[7] A critical filter had been inadvertently left out of the X-ray machine when the treatment was administered, and the damage to the child's scalp was almost immediately evident. Within weeks he developed ulcers on his scalp which would not heal, and his hair began to fall out. In time, it was evident that the damage was permanent and might develop further into still more serious consequences.

The Lovelace authorities had immediately accepted full responsibility for the accident,[8] and they tried all possible means of treating the child's problems locally. When that failed, the clinic sent the patient and his family to the Mayo Clinic for consultation, and over the first few years after the accident, the institution spent more than 20,000 dollars in trying to help the injured boy. All efforts at settlement of the family's grievance outside court failed, and in 1966, eight years after the original accident, the Lucas family filed a 2.3-million-dollar damage suit against the Lovelace Clinic in district court.[9] The case dragged through the legal process for another two years before it was finally heard in the spring of 1968. The clinic expected to lose, but it was assured by its attorneys that the highest judgment on record in New Mexico was the 400,000 dollars paid to a child who had lost both parents and had been crippled in an auto accident caused by a drunken driver. The clinic's malpractice insurance afforded coverage of 100,000 dollars for each of its staff members or employees; and since three staff members had been involved in treatment of the Lucas child, even the most severe judgment possible did not threaten to become intoler-

7. Lovelace Clinic, Board of Governors, Minutes, 30 January 1968; the Lawrence Lucas file, Lovelace Medical Center archives.

8. It later developed that the manufacturer of the X-ray equipment used in the treatment of the Lucas child had been sued at least twice in other states on charges of negligence in failing to furnish protective devices to guard against just such accidental exposures as in the Lucas case; but since there were no charges of product liability in this case, the Lovelace Clinic never succeeded in recovering any compensation from the manufacturer. Lovelace Clinic, Board of Governors, Minutes, 25 February 1969 and 5 August 1969.

9. For samples of the damaging press coverage of the case, see *Albuquerque Tribune*, 7 April 1966, and both the *Albuquerque Journal* and *Albuquerque Tribune* for April and May 1968.

ably damaging financially to the institution. When the Lucas case jury rendered its verdict on 25 April 1968—1.25 million dollars to be paid to the Lucas family by the clinic—the Lovelace institution was shaken to its core, and the southwestern medical community was shocked.[10] It was an unimaginable situation, but its reality was brought home in the most tangible way on Tuesday, 30 April 1968, when a deputy sheriff arrived at the clinic's business office with a signed execution order requesting immediate payment of 950,000 dollars plus expenses.

Robert O. Anderson, chairman of the Lovelace Foundation since the preceding year, intervened personally on the clinic's behalf to assure the court of the Lovelace authorities' intention to satisfy the judgment; thus, the formal padlocking of the clinic—a realistic possibility—was averted. Over subsequent weeks, a settlement with the Lucas family was worked out, and Anderson and other trustee-friends of the Lovelace enterprise arranged for the money to pay the settlement. However, the unpleasant publicity associated with the case was compromising to the clinic's reputation, and rumors regarding the development and meaning of the case and its possible consequences upset the normal equilibrium of the institution. Before the quick and efficacious intervention by Anderson and the colleagues he enlisted in the clinic's cause, there was grave uncertainty and anxiety within the complex on Gibson Boulevard.[11] The furor over the episode eventually waned without permanent harm to the institution, but it contributed to the sense of uncertainty, even fragility, felt during the transitional years following the departure of the founders from the scene.

In the summer of 1970, Dr. Grossman, with his energies sapped by the unwanted responsibilities of running the clinic, resigned his post as chairman of its board and was succeeded by another staff veteran, Dr. Donald E. Kilgore, Jr. An otolar-

10. Lovelace Clinic, Board of Governors, Minutes, 30 January 1968.

11. The private correspondence of eighty-four-year-old Dr. Lovelace reflected the dimensions of the worry within the medical center. In a letter to a physician friend he wrote, "We are having some serious difficulties at the clinic with a suit that has been brought against us for a mistake that was made by one of the X-ray technicians. I am greatly disturbed over it." Dr. William Randolph Lovelace I, to Dr. James Walker Ralph, 2 May 1968.

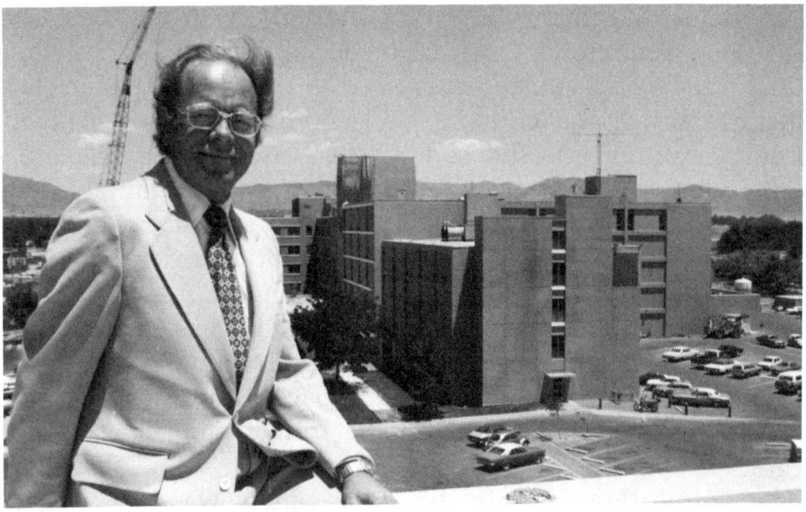

Dr. Donald E. Kilgore, in 1975, with a part of the Lovelace Medical Center he served as president and chief executive officer in the background.

yngologist with twenty years of experience at Lovelace—a former navy flier, he had been attracted to the clinic in 1953 by its concentration in aviation medicine—Dr. Kilgore had risen to a position of influence within the institution in the years following Randy Lovelace's death. First elected to the Board of Governors in early 1965, Dr. Kilgore was devoted to the Lovelace center and its principles and objectives. Like Dr. Grossman before him, he did not so much seek power as have it thrust upon him. An extremely capable and decisive man, Dr. Kilgore had caught the eye of Lovelace Foundation Chairman Robert O. Anderson in the late sixties; and Anderson's support, combined with the general respect and confidence that Kilgore enjoyed within the clinic's staff, produced his elevation to the post of cochairman (with Dr. Grossman) of the clinic's Board of Governors in January 1970, and then to the chairmanship in August, when Dr. Grossman resigned.

Serious problems immediately confronted Dr. Kilgore when he took over leadership of the Lovelace institution. Most obvious of all was the glaring need for professionalization of the center's administration. The Clinic, in particular, was run as a kind of "cottage industry", and there was no apparent interest or commitment to modernization of its operations. One contemporary observer noted caustically, "the Trustees chose to keep it that way while they hoped that a messiah would emerge to fill Randy's shoes, but no such messiah was forthcoming."[12] While Dr. Kilgore worked to establish some degree of professional administration within the Lovelace center, it was additionally his unhappy fate to have to wrestle with the gravest financial crisis that had ever confronted the Lovelace Clinic; and there were moments in 1973 and 1974 when the very future of the proud institution seemed to be in doubt. (The full dimensions of the difficulties are agonizingly clear in the minutes of the 23 October 1973 meeting of the clinic's Board of Governors, as Dr. Kilgore told his glum colleagues "that the last payroll had been in jeopardy of not being met" and that local banks had refused to extend to the clinic any further credit.)[13]

These acute money difficulties were the product of a number of different forces. The basic problem was the necessity for refinancing the institution to enable it to handle the much expanded responsibilities it had accepted during the years of its rapid growth and development. By 1970, the income available to the center was simply inadequate for the institution's purposes, and its Board of Trustees was reluctant to accept the unavoidability of refinancing. One specific difficulty was the gradual inflation of the nonmedical staff over the years, producing costs that were increasingly difficult to bear. Another problem lay in the fact that some clinic physicians had lost their zest for practice, for various reasons, and were being carried to a large degree by their more productive colleagues. In addition, the institution was woefully undercapitalized at the very time that it was faced with rapidly escalating equipment costs and the potpourri of problems associated with an aging physical plant. Administrative worries compounded the situation, chief

12. Private communication.

13. Lovelace Clinic, Board of Governors, Minutes, 23 October 1973. For the eight-month period from October 1973 through May 1974, the hemorrhage continued as the clinic lost another 315,000 dollars despite paying no rent during that time. Lovelace Clinic, Board of Governors, Minutes, 18 June 1974.

among them the inability of the clinic's business office to cope with a deepening accounts-receivables problem; by 1974, collections were running 120 days late and beyond. External factors also conspired to make the clinic's economic challenge more formidable in the early 1970s. For example, the clinic had tried to keep its charges low throughout the late 1960s and now found itself locked into those low-end charges by the price-control measures initiated by the Nixon administration in the early seventies. Also, the competitive environment in Albuquerque noticeably grew more fierce in the late sixties and seventies as the city's private-practice community increased in numbers and in the sophistication of its skills, and as the new University of New Mexico Medical School and the Presbyterian Hospital system, in particular, grew remarkably as competitors to the Lovelace center.

One of the most damaging consequences of the worsening financial picture at the clinic was a significant rise in the physician-turnover rate at the institution. Of course, there had always been a moderate measure of turnover of the Lovelace staff, as physicians decided that they did not like group practice, or preferred some other locale, and simply wanted to try their hands at solo practice with its (usually) higher earnings. Over the years, the Lovelace Clinic had perhaps a slightly higher turnover rate than normal, primarily because of Uncle Doc's penuriousness with salary and with power. However, the turnover rate of the early seventies was exceptional, and from August 1971 to October 1973 the clinic lost twenty-seven staff members—roughly 20 percent each year—some through retirement, but most simply moving on to more lucrative situations. Some doctors involved in that exodus were sincerely concerned about the long-term viability of the institution; others were simply taking advantage of the elimination of the restrictive covenant clause; but almost all of them were convinced that they were badly underpaid and could earn much more outside the clinic. The rapid turnover intensified the clinic's financial woes, for many of those who departed had well-established reputations and practices that were lost to the clinic, and it cost considerable sums of money to recruit and to try to establish replacements. In addition to the financial costs, the departure of so many staff members within such a short period of time contributed to the steady erosion of morale within the institution. The clinic's staff, which had been generally stable at sixty-five to seventy physicians during the late sixties, eventually fell to fifty-two in mid-1976.

The situation was not helped by the development of a growing rift, from 1973 to 1975, between Dr. Kilgore and the clinic's medical director, Dr. Frank Mowry. Dr. Mowry, a well-trained and passionately dedicated cardiologist who had first come to the clinic in 1965, was elected medical director of the group practice in September 1972, and he quickly began determined efforts to improve the caliber of medical practice, as he saw it, within the Lovelace staff. Programmatic and philosophical differences of opinion tended to separate the ambitious and sometimes impatient cardiologist and Dr. Kilgore, and personal differences in style added to the tension developing between them. Substantive disagreements between the two leaders about the future of Lovelace's pioneering health-maintenance organization (see pp. 174–181) and about the handling of the medical staff eventually provoked an open breach in the fall of 1975, a confrontation that was finally resolved by the resignation of both men.[14]

One of the most important measures undertaken by Dr. Kilgore as chairman of the Lovelace Clinic was aimed specifically at reducing the overall costs of operations on the Lovelace campus and, beyond that, at tighter, more effective coordination of the several health-related enterprises on Gibson Boulevard. This was the merger of all disparate elements of the Lovelace operations into one entity called the Lovelace-Bataan Medical Center. The merger process, which stretched from 1969 to 1973, is properly associated with Dr. Kilgore, who devoted great chunks of his limited time[15] and energy to that effort. Years after the fact, Dr. Kilgore remembered that achievement as his most important assignment:

14. Dr. Mowry left the staff of the clinic for private practice in Albuquerque, while Dr. Kilgore returned to full-time clinical practice and leadership of the clinic's Department of Otolaryngology. As of 1986, his thirty-three years on the Lovelace staff made him second in seniority among its members, surpassed only by Dr. Tom Chiffelle, clinic pathologist, who had come to Lovelace a year earlier.

15. One of the special difficulties of the Kilgore administration was Dr. Kilgore's insistence on keeping up a major portion of his clinical practice, often as much as six hours or more a day.

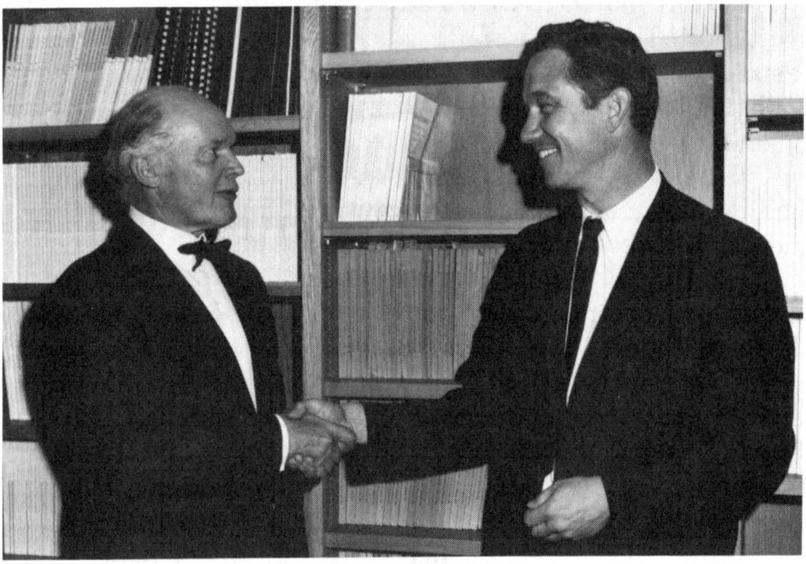

Robert O. Anderson, chairman of the board of the Lovelace Medical Foundation, is shown at left in this photograph with Joe R. G. Fulcher, longtime administrator and legal counsellor to the foundation.

> My principal objective when I assumed the chairmanship of the Board of Governors was to get all these institutions under one banner. We had five different corporations going, something like 32 different insurance policies covering the institution, duplicate this and triplicate that, different boards—Board of Directors of the Hospital, Board of Trustees of the Foundation, Board of Governors of the Clinic, and so on. It made things awkward to the point of impossibility in terms of getting anything done.[16]

The other key figure in inspiring and supporting the merger process until it was completed was the new (as of 1967) chairman of the Lovelace Foundation's Board of Trustees: oilman, businessman, and rancher Robert O. Anderson. This adopted New Mexican and world-renowned business leader was perhaps the central figure in the Lovelace institution's history from

16. Kilgore, interview, 18 November 1985.

the end of the sixties until the end of the eighties, playing a central and personal role in its development. Anderson, a powerhouse in the domestic oil industry and one of the largest landowners in the nation, provided indispensable counsel, contacts, and financial assistance to the Lovelace center over the quarter-century of his association with it, and he gave it large measures of his hard-pressed time and energies. He first became connected with the Albuquerque institution through his personal friendship with Randy Lovelace. After the latter's death, Anderson remained close because of his belief in the institution and its mission and because of his pride in what this native-born institution had achieved.[17] Anderson had made much of his reputation in the oil business by skillfully putting small units together to make larger ones, and it was he who inspired and encouraged Dr. Kilgore throughout the merger process on the Lovelace campus. He initiated the merger in 1968, the year after he succeeded Floyd Odlum as chairman of the foundation board, by urging Lovelace authorities to contract for a professional management survey of the structure and operations of the center. That outside evaluation, accomplished by the New York management consultant firm Cresap, McCormick and Paget early in the spring of 1969, recommended significant changes in the Lovelace organization. While the professionals lauded the accomplishments of the Albuquerque institution over the brief twenty years since the 1947 reorganization and reorientation directed by Randy Lovelace, they also insisted emphatically on the need for and stressed the many advantages to be obtained by tighter coordination and management of the Gibson complex.[18]

The report of the prestigious management consultants, coupled with Chairman Anderson's assurance of financial help, crystallized a growing consensus inside the Lovelace center about the need for rationalization of its structure and business

17. Robert O. Anderson, interview with the author, Albuquerque, 30 August 1985.

18. Cresap, McCormick and Paget, Inc., "Lovelace Foundation for Medical Education and Research, Lovelace Clinic, Bataan Memorial Methodist Hospital: A Reconnaissance Review of Organization and Management" (typescript), 4 March 1969, in Lovelace Medical Center archives.

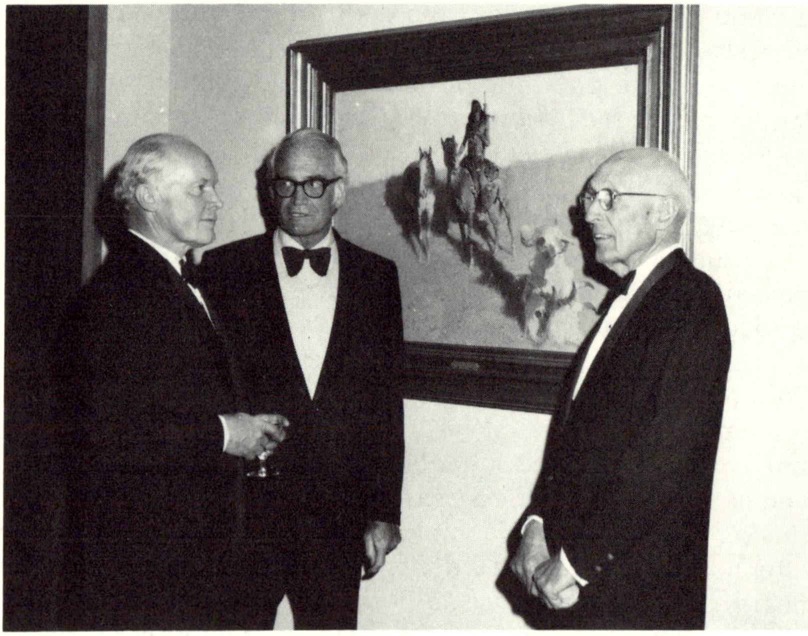

Robert O. Anderson, left, and Albert Mitchell, right, greet Senator Barry Goldwater of Arizona, who gave the fourth W. Randolph Lovelace II Memorial Lecture in 1972. The men stand before one of the western art masterpieces that Mr. Mitchell loaned for display at the Lovelace center.

practices, and the first step forward was taken in late 1969 with the purchase of Bataan Memorial Methodist Hospital by the Lovelace Foundation.

The 223-bed, full-service general hospital was owned in 1969 by the New Mexico Annual Conference of the Methodist Church. (Ownership of the hospital had been transferred in 1965 from the original owners, the Methodist Church Women's Society of Christian Service, to the local authorities.) It had an open staff policy, and more than 229 active and courtesy staff physicians were on its rolls in 1968, but over 84 percent of its more than 8,500 patients in 1968 were admitted by Lovelace Clinic physicians.[19] During the late 1960s, the hospital consistently

19. Bataan Memorial Methodist Hospital, *Annual Report, 1968*, p. 14.

ran small deficits which were covered by funds from the church's annual conference. Though small, the deficits were worrisome, for the church's budget was already strained by the demands of its operational budget and the pension requirements of the many retired ministers and other church workers for whom it was responsible. Since Bataan Hospital represented a considerable sum of "locked-in" capital, which might be put to more productive use elsewhere, the church authorities were interested in selling their property.[20] Negotiations with authorities of the Lovelace Foundation produced an offer of two million dollars in cash for the hospital—Chairman Anderson personally pledged 1.6 million dollars toward the acquisition—and the deal was struck. On 31 October 1969, the hospital became a part of the Lovelace Foundation, and the first major step toward consolidation was accomplished. The fusion of the clinic and the hospital was far more difficult, since it involved combination of a professional association and a nonprofit institution; but that merger was also engineered in complex negotiations and precise legal procedures spanning 1971 and 1972. On 4 January 1973, the clinic and hospital were fused in a new nonprofit, tax-exempt health-care corporation called the Lovelace Center for the Health Sciences; and because the new center's Board of Trustees and officers interlocked with those of the Lovelace Foundation for Medical Education and Research (see Table 6), the union of the health care complex was complete.[21] Through the remainder of 1973, all departments common to the clinic, foundation, hospital, nursing home, and health program[22] were

20. Horace McKay, interview with the author, Albuquerque, 9 December 1985. McKay, a prominent lay member of the hospital board, was a crucial link to the Lovelace Foundation. With the full support and assistance of Bishop Alsie H. Carleton of the Methodist Church, McKay helped to negotiate the sale.

21. The details of the merger, too intricate and esoteric for consideration here, may be traced through the annual reports of the foundation and the minutes and documents of the clinic's Board of Governors. The legal process was brilliantly orchestrated by Joe R. G. Fulcher, a lawyer and longtime administrator of the foundation. See Joe R. G. Fulcher, interview with the author, Albuquerque, 11 December 1986, for more details and the "feel" of the merger.

22. In 1964 the Lovelace Foundation had purchased the 96-bed Ridgecrest Manor nursing home, located on land adjacent to Lovelace property, and ran the nursing home as a division of its overall operations.

Table 6 Board of Trustees, Lovelace-Bataan Medical Center, 1973

Robert O. Anderson, *Roswell, New Mexico. Industrialist and Rancher, Chairman of the Board, Atlantic Richfield Company*

Sherburne P. Anderson, *Albuquerque, New Mexico. President, Clinton P. Anderson Agency, Incorporated.*

Robert H. Beck, *Roswell, New Mexico. Publisher, Roswell Daily Record.*

Cale W. Carson, Jr., *Albuquerque, New Mexico. President, First National Bank in Albuquerque.*

Oliver S. Cramer, M.D., *Albuquerque, New Mexico. Physician, retired.*

J. Leslie Davis, *Cimarron, New Mexico. Rancher.*

Alvin C. Eurich, Ph.D., *New York, New York. President, Academy for Educational Development, Incorporated.*

Joe R. G. Fulcher, *Albuquerque, New Mexico. Attorney-at-Law.*

Jack J. Hall, *Chicago, Illinois. President, J.J. Hall Enterprises.*

A. E. Johnson, *Denver, Colorado. Chairman of the Board, Midwest Oil Corporation.*

Earl D. Johnson, *Greenwich, Connecticut. Aviation Consultant.*

H. Mikkel Kelly, *Albuquerque, New Mexico. Hospital Executive.*

Donald E. Kilgore, Jr., M.D., *Albuquerque, New Mexico. Chief Executive Officer, Physician and Surgeon, Lovelace-Bataan Medical Center.*

Jack A. Korber, *Albuquerque, New Mexico. Owner, J. Korber & Company.*

E. L. Lassetter, M.D., *Albuquerque, New Mexico. Physician, Lovelace-Bataan Medical Center.*

Robert S. LeSage, *Dallas, Tex. Rancher and Investments.*

Oscar M. Love, *Albuquerque, New Mexico. Co-Chairman of the Board and President Emeritus, Albuquerque National Bank.*

Oscar Mahlon Love, Jr., *Albuquerque, New Mexico. Vice-President, Albuquerque National Bank.*

Frank A. Mapel, *Albuquerque, New Mexico. President, Coca-Cola Bottling Company of Durango, Colorado and Farmington, New Mexico.*

Jack D. McCarthy, M.D., *Albuquerque, New Mexico. Physician and Surgeon, Lovelace-Bataan Medical Center.*

Horace F. McKay, Jr., *Albuquerque, New Mexico. Investments.*

D. Angus McKinnon, Jr., M.D., *Albuquerque, New Mexico. Physician and Surgeon, Lovelace-Bataan Medical Center.*

J. T. Michelson, *Albuquerque, New Mexico. President, Sunbell Corporation.*

Albert K. Mitchell, *Albert, New Mexico. Rancher.*

Sidney Salomon, Jr., *St. Louis, Missouri. Insurance Broker.*

C. R. Smith, *New York, New York. Chairman and Chief Executive Officer, Board of Directors, American Airlines.*

Harold Stuart, *Vice-President, Tulsa, Oklahoma. Attorney and Corporation Executive.*

Robert S. Turner, M.D., *Albuquerque, New Mexico. Physician and Surgeon, Lovelace-Bataan Medical Center.*

William Thayer Tutt, *Colorado Springs, Colorado. President, The Broadmoor Hotel Corporation.*

Ulf S. von Euler, M.D., *Stockholm, Sweden. Professor Emeritus, Karolinska Institute, Nobel Laureate.*

Clayton S. White, M.D., *Albuquerque, New Mexico. President-Director and Director of Research, Lovelace Foundation for Medical Education and Research.*

Lord Zuckerman, *of Burnham Thorpe. Professor at Large, University of East Anglia, Norwich, England.*

EMERITUS

David G. Baird, *New York, New York. Financier.*

Floyd B. Odlum, *Indio, California. Financier and Rancher; Chairman Emeritus, Lovelace Foundation for Medical Education and Research.*

Vernon J. Pick, *Denver, Colorado. Owner, Pick Enterprises.*

Robert C. Reeve, *Anchorage, Alaska. President, Reeve Aleutian Airways, Incorporated.*

Louis J. Reynolds, *Santa Fe, New Mexico. Investments.*

EXECUTIVE COMMITTEE
Donald E. Kilgore, Jr., M.D., *Chairman*

Robert O. Anderson	Horace F. McKay, Jr.
Sherburne P. Anderson	D. Angus McKinnon, Jr., M.D.
Jack A. Korber	Albert K. Mitchell
Oscar M. Love	Clayton S. White, M.D.
Frank P. Mapel	

LOVELACE CENTER FOR THE HEALTH SCIENCES	OFFICERS	LOVELACE FOUNDATION FOR MEDICAL EDUCATION & RESEARCH
Chairman, Board of Trustees	Robert O. Anderson	*Chairman, Board of Trustees*
Vice Chairman, Board of Trustees; Chairman, Executive Committee; President and Chief Executive Officer	Donald E. Kilgore, Jr., M.D.	*Vice Chairman, Board of Trustees; Chairman, Executive Committee; and Chief Executive Officer*
Chairman Emeritus	Floyd B. Odlum	*Chairman Emeritus*
	Clayton S. White, M.D.	*President-Director*
Vice President	Horace F. McKay, Jr.	*Vice President*
	Roger O. McClellan, DVM	*Vice President and Director of Research Administration*
Secretary	Jack A. Korber	*Secretary*
Treasurer	Sherburne P. Anderson	*Treasurer*

consolidated in an orderly fashion, and improvements in the economy and efficiency of operations were quickly evident.

The merger of the various organizations on the Lovelace campus had a remarkable salutary effect on the institution's operations and its capacity for adaptation, planning, and development; but it did not help immediately in resolution of the problems growing within the clinic. Throughout 1974 and 1975, the precarious financial position of the group practice and the continued exodus of staff physicians claimed far more attention than the prosaic, if ultimately far more important, reorganization and consolidation work inherent in the merger process and the initial planning of brave new ventures for the future. Thus, the years of the early 1970s are often remembered solely as a "time of troubles" on Gibson Boulevard; in actuality, however, there was also much of long-term and positive significance under way. The successful execution of the merger challenge was only one example. It was also the Kilgore administration that set up the Lovelace center's pioneering health maintenance organization (HMO); initiated its satellite operations, which proved so beneficial to the center's long-range health; and began the reorientation or reemphasis within the institution on primary care. Nevertheless, it was time in 1975 for new leadership, and Chairman Anderson presided over a nationwide search for a new chief executive. The committee sought a progressive physician-executive who would provide stability and clear direction as the Lovelace Medical Center confronted the rapidly changing health-care environment of the last quarter of the twentieth century.

The new leader was found in Dr. David J. Ottensmeyer, a forty-five-year-old neurosurgeon who had been president and chief executive officer of Wisconsin's large and innovative Marshfield Clinic from 1972 to 1975. Dr. Ottensmeyer, a step ahead of most of his colleagues, already possessed the rare blend of medical and managerial talent and the training essential for success in the much more complex and competitive medical world of the seventies and eighties. His medical background was impeccable—medical school at the University of Wisconsin and a residency there in neurological surgery, followed by a decade of clinical practice at the Marshfield (Wisconsin) Clinic—but early in his career he had shown great interest in and a flair for medical administration. At Marshfield he was increasingly active in the clinic's governance, and quickly rose from its vice presidency to become its president and chief executive officer after a scant seven years on the scene. He formally studied health-services management through a special program of the Harvard Business School in 1975, and later earned an M.S. degree in Health Care Administration from St. Francis College in Illinois. When interviewed for the top spot at Lovelace in the spring of 1976, he was immediately impressed by its achievements and by the caliber of people who supported the place. Its problems were readily apparent as well, but on balance he was more impressed by its prospects. When the job of president and chief executive officer was offered to him, he accepted and arrived on the scene in Albuquerque at about the time of the nation's bicentennial celebrations.[23]

23. For his impressions of the Lovelace center in 1976 and his analysis of its strengths and weaknesses, see Dr. David J. Ottensmeyer, interview with the author, Albuquerque, 23 August 1985 and passim.

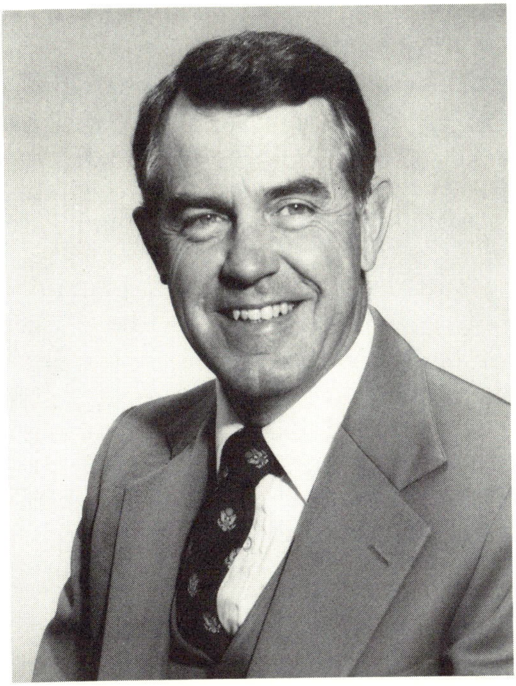

Dr. David J. Ottensmeyer, president and chief executive officer of the Lovelace Medical Center from 1976 to 1986.

Because the Lovelace Clinic remained the key to the overall health and well-being of the Lovelace Medical Center, and since its problems were the most immediate and threatening, Dr. Ottensmeyer first turned his attention and energies there. Two broad and basic problems were at the top of his agenda. First, efforts had to be made immediately to reverse the paralyzing decline in numbers and morale within the ranks of the clinic's physicians. Recovery to full health of the medical staff was the indispensable first step toward revival of the clinic's fortunes. Second, the expenses of the center's operations needed renewed scrutiny, especially its relatively high personnel outlays; for cuts in expenditures were required immediately as a step toward restoring financial stability to the center. In focusing on these priorities, the new chief executive spent his first few months in Albuquerque recruiting new physicians and seeking means of improving conditions for those already in the organization. Recruiting took much of his time, but it paid handsome dividends. By the end of 1976 he had already hired ten new physicians—most of them bright, energetic young doctors fresh from strong residency programs—and seven more were due to arrive over the next few months. This rebuilding of the clinic's staff capabilities—as Uncle Doc had known so well, patient volume was the key to a successful group practice—continued through the first two years of the Ottensmeyer tenure; then, staff size stabilized for a few years at the level of seventy-five to eighty-five physicians representing more than two dozen specialties and subspecialties. It did not prove difficult to persuade talented young doctors to come to Lovelace, despite its financial shakiness, for its problems were largely invisible while the center itself remained a large and impressive institution.[24] Furthermore, a second element in Dr. Ottensmeyer's plan for restoring the clinic's medical staff to full strength and vigor involved raising the salary levels of Lovelace physicians at least to national norms.

Salaries had been a perennial problem through the half-century of the clinic's history down to 1976. The salary question had certainly played a major role in the exodus of physicians in the early seventies. In 1972, Medical Director Mowry and the clinic's Board of Governors had tried to do something about the problem by instituting a new salary program which gave less emphasis to seniority than previously and more to productivity; but Lovelace salaries continued to lag behind the average for group practices as well as behind community standards.[25] Dr. Ottensmeyer immediately announced his objective of raising physician salaries to at least the fiftieth percentile nationally, and followed the announcement with a round of

24. Interviews with several of the young doctors hired from 1976 to 1978 emphasized this point. See, for example, the interview with Dr. Mel Twiest (interview with the author, Albuquerque, 22 September 1986 and passim). The young surgeon remembered being highly impressed with the visible strength of the Lovelace complex, especially (for him) its beautiful, large library.

25. Available evidence suggests that Lovelace salaries were roughly 10 to 15 percent below the national norms for group practices, and much testimony—most of it slippery—indicates that they were below community averages as well.

salary increases in January 1977, "even though the money wasn't really there yet."[26] New doctors were hired at nationally competitive scales, and over the decade of Dr. Ottensmeyer's tenure at Lovelace, salaries rose to levels fully competitive both nationally and locally. The effect on staff morale was predictable, and as morale improved so did productivity. The staff retention rate quickly reflected the change, and by the mid-1980s the turnover yearly at Lovelace had sunk to about 5 percent.

But Dr. Ottensmeyer's plans for strengthening the medical staff of the clinic included more than simply expanding its numbers and enhancing its stability and morale through better salaries. The reorganization he sought called for a much more extensive and intimate involvement by the doctors in the management of the Lovelace medical center. The argument could be made that the Lovelace Clinic had never been a true group practice, with members of the group collegially responsible for its direction and management. The Albuquerque group had very definitely been Uncle Doc's clinic up to 1947; then, Randy Lovelace had taken control, benignly and beneficently, with his uncle in the background, until his death in 1965. The decade prior to Dr. Ottensmeyer's arrival had seen some tentative movement toward increasing physician participation in directing the affairs of the center, but that progress had been interrupted by the merger process and the acute financial problems of the early seventies, both of which tended to bring laymen of the Board of Trustees into more direct managerial and planning roles than before. To a considerable degree, the issues of the early seventies had shunted the physicians of the group to the sideline.[27] Dr. Ottensmeyer operated on the premise that the Lovelace medical complex could cope most efficiently in the increasingly competitive world of corporate medicine only if it could "come to grips with the medical staff by integrating it centrally everywhere in the operation."[28] To both the veterans

26. Ottensmeyer, interview, 23 August 1985.

27. This was reflected, Dr. Ottensmeyer thought, in the fact that when he first came to Lovelace for an interview in March 1976, he did not meet a single physician until well into his second day in town. Ottensmeyer, interview, 23 August 1985.

28. Ibid.

of the organization and to the new physicians he recruited, he emphasized that Lovelace's new leadership was dedicated to a set of values that recognized the centrality of the medical group within the institution's operations.[29] As a concrete sign of that commitment, in September 1976—a scant three months after his arrival to head the Albuquerque center—Dr. Ottensmeyer persuaded the pivotally important executive committee of the organization to consider fundamental reform in the governance of the center. He called on this standing committee of the Board of Trustees, charged with control of the institution in its name, to initiate a quick but thorough study of the "role of the medical staff and its involvement in decision making at the level of the Board of Trustees."[30] At that time, the executive committee's makeup reflected the weakness of physician influence at the center; it was composed of seven laymen and two physicians of the Lovelace medical staff. As a result of the reexamination requested and inspired by Dr. Ottensmeyer, the trustees of the Lovelace medical center met in special session in November 1976 to approve changes in the bylaws of the center, which reconstituted the executive committee by placing the five physicians of the clinic's Board of Governors on the committee, along with six other trustees (who might also be physicians); thus, a new eleven-member group, with far stronger physician input in its deliberations, was created.[31] Following this reform, the influence of the clinic's physicians has been far more central in the operation of the entire medical center, even though some critics have argued that Dr. Ottensmeyer's leadership was so strong and his success so quick and striking that the institution's doctors were largely content simply to follow his lead.[32]

29. Ottensmeyer, interview, 23 August 1985.

30. Lovelace Center for the Health Sciences, *Annual Report*, 1976, p. 3.

31. Lovelace Foundation for Medical Education and Research, Board of Trustees, Minutes, 8 November 1976.

32. The position paper of one (successful) candidate for the clinic's Board of Governors in 1982—and thus for a seat on the institution's executive committee as well—worried, "The direction of this organization at this time is basically attributable to one individual, and laudable though his efforts and achievements may be, I do not believe that this is a healthy situation." Lovelace Medical Center, Medical Staff, Minutes, November 1982.

Structurally, however, the governmental reform of late 1976 and the invigoration of the clinic's Board of Governors, which was so basic a part of it, gave the medical staff more integral decision-making authority than ever before. This change, too, contributed to a renewed confidence and sense of participation within the ranks of the center's pivotally important physicians. However, new responsibilities for the physicians were associated with this reform. It was the conviction of the Ottensmeyer administration that, if the staff's doctors were to assume greater managerial authority within the institution, then they needed to prepare themselves appropriately through formal study of modern management and health care administration. During the 1980s, the Lovelace medical center became a national leader in requiring high standards of training for its modern physician-managers.

Almost simultaneously, Dr. Ottensmeyer undertook a full-scale study of staffing levels at the center. It was obvious that the size of the support staff at the medical center had swollen significantly with the passage of time—which was to be expected with the growth of the organization—but there had been very little direct administrative supervision or control over the process. As a result, by the end of 1973 the employees of the Lovelace medical complex numbered nearly 1,400, with the clinic paying 553 people, the foundation 269, and the hospital another 555.[33] At that time, efforts were initiated to control and to alleviate the problem, and those endeavors, in addition to a large measure of natural attrition, had already shrunk the payroll to some 1,150 by the time of the new chief executive's arrival. The reduction process had trimmed away most of the organization's excess, and thus, Dr. Ottensmeyer's January 1977 announcement of the layoff of an additional 188 full-time employees cut perilously close to the bone. In reporting the measure to the medical staff, he insisted that his studies justified the action—comparable group practices around the nation average thirteen employees for each physician, while the ratio at Lovelace was sixteen to one—but he also argued that the layoff

33. Lovelace Clinic, Board of Governors, Minutes, 23 October 1973.

was imperative in terms of economic necessity. The action would save the center approximately 12,000 dollars per employee, thus more than 2 million dollars in one year alone.[34] This first layoff in the institution's history was hardly a pleasant move, but it was essential to the financial health of the organization, stripping the Lovelace complex down to fighting trim as it began the task of reestablishing its financial strength.

The reforms of the first few months of the Ottensmeyer administration had both immediate and long-term significance, but it was the combination of three other major developments of the late seventies which decisively set the Lovelace center back on its feet and on the road toward a position of authority locally as well as nationally. Key elements in the powerful resurgence of the Lovelace center during the 1980s were the reorientation of the clinic's philosophy to include a strong emphasis on primary care; the blossoming of New Mexico's pioneering and most successful health-maintenance organization; and the construction of a chain of satellite clinics scattered around the city, which took the Lovelace Clinic where the people were.

Primary care in the sense of the old general practitioner or family doctor, who treated his patients for minor ills and referred them to specialists when circumstances required it, had always been a part of the Lovelace tradition. It was certainly the type of practice that Uncle Doc Lovelace and Ed Lassetter had served in building the Lovelace Clinic. Even into the early fifties, long after the effort to make the Lovelace Clinic a center of specialty medicine was under way, there was a good deal of blurring of specialty lines. If a patient came to the Lovelace Clinic and wanted to see Dr. Randy Lovelace specifically, he usually got his wish. The surgeon would see him, listen to the problem, perhaps take a brief history, and then treat the patient or refer him to someone whose skills were clearly more relevant to the particular case.[35] Throughout the fifties and sixties, however, the thrust within the clinic was distinctly toward specialty

34. Lovelace Center for the Health Sciences, Medical Staff, Minutes, 14 February 1977.

35. Dr. Clayton S. White, interview with the author, Albuquerque, 14 October 1985 and passim.

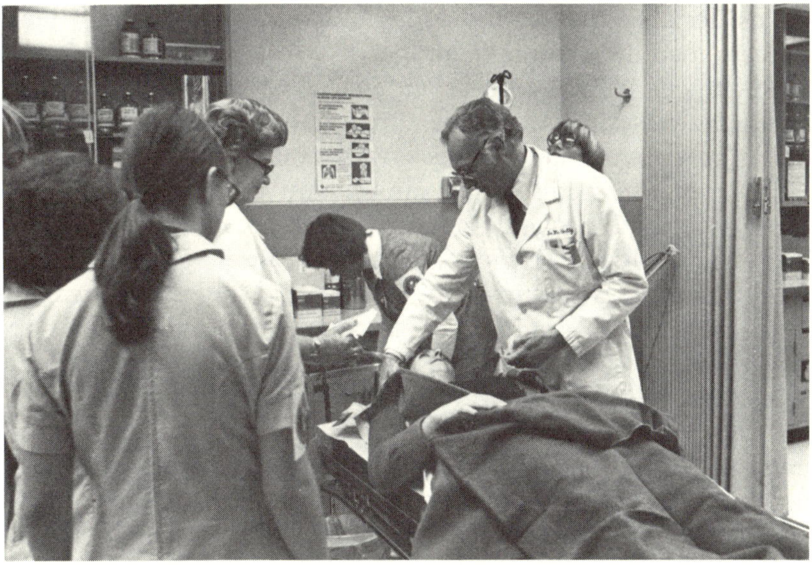

Dr. Jack McCarthy, twenty-five-year veteran of the clinic staff and head of its Department of General Surgery, examines a patient. Dr. McCarthy served as chairman of the clinic's Board of Governors in the transitional period between the administrations of Drs. Kilgore and Ottensmeyer.

medicine, with Lovelace specialists providing secondary and tertiary care to patients referred by community or regional physicians or to patients attracted by the clinic's name. The conviction inherent in that allegiance to specialty medicine (and the slight, but unmistakable, sense of superiority associated with it) was reflected in the experience of Dr. Donald Kilgore when he arrived at the clinic in 1953. At that time, the young physician was devoted to the idea of family practice, a term not yet in common usage; but his lack of specialty qualifications disturbed some of his specialist-colleagues. One of them, Dr. Lee Monroe Miles, a clinic veteran of twenty years and head of its Obstetrics-Gynecology Department, called Kilgore into his office one day to tell him frankly that although he was a fine young man and undoubtedly would become an excellent doctor, he really had no place at a high-powered, multispecialty group practice such as the Lovelace Clinic; in particular, Dr.

Miles declared that he did not want "family medicine" practitioners meddling in his field.[36]

By the early 1970s, however, an exclusive focus on specialty medicine was far more problematic than earlier. For one thing, the differentiation and increasing sophistication of Albuquerque's private-practice physicians meant that the clinic's specialists were no longer unique within the community.[37] There were relatively few services available at the clinic that could not be secured elsewhere in Albuquerque; and there was a realistic concern that solo practitioners in the community, if they were given the choice between referring to specialists in private practice or those at the clinic, would almost always prefer the former. (It was conventional wisdom that a private practitioner referring a patient to the clinic ran the risk that the patient might choose to seek all of his care there.) Without a primary-care base for referrals to the center, Lovelace specialty medicine might suffer seriously for lack of patients. This reexamination of the role of primary care within the Lovelace system was encouraged by the 1969 Cresap, McCormick, and Paget study of the center, which showed that a full 91.1 percent of all patients visiting the clinic in 1967 were Albuquerqueans (63.0 percent) or were from elsewhere in New Mexico (28.1 percent). For many on Gibson Boulevard, the logic of these statistics was inescapable. Since the clinic already was, in fact, a community group practice—and not a so-called magnet clinic like the Mayo or Cleveland clinics, which attracted most of their patients from elsewhere—why not focus on that market and provide all the health-care consumer's needs, rather than catering to his occasional need for specialty medicine? Further, a strong primary care capability would undoubtedly strengthen Lovelace specialty medicine practice through internal referrals.

What some call Lovelace's "first push into primary care" began then, in the early 1970s. Orchestrated largely by Medical

36. Kilgore, interview, 18 November 1985.

37. On the development of specialty medicine in Albuquerque and throughout New Mexico, see Jake W. Spidle, Jr., *Doctors of Medicine in New Mexico: A History of Health and Medical Practice, 1886–1986* (Albuquerque: University of New Mexico Press, 1986), pp. 294–98.

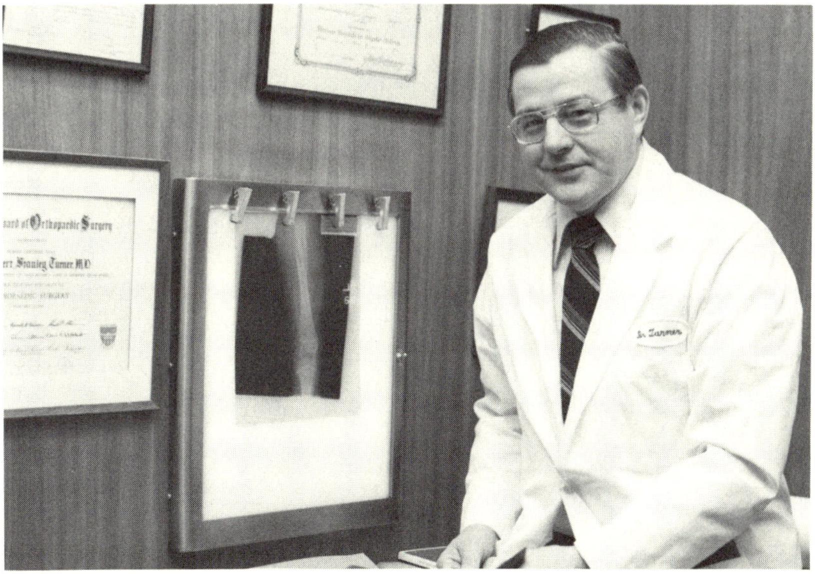

Dr. Robert S. Turner, head of the clinic's orthopaedic surgery department, gave more than a quarter century of service to the Lovelace center and played a key role in the clinic's leadership in the late 1960s and 1970s.

Director Mowry, it took the form of hiring increased numbers of board-certified general internists and pediatricians to act as the primary-care providers for the entire system. The new policy was only marginally successful, for board-certified internists and pediatricians proved not to be the most cost-effective providers of primary care, and they were not always broad enough in their range of practice to fill that role. More seriously, the clinic's primary-care capacity was not where the people were. In the 1970s, as Albuquerque's west mesa, far northeast heights, and then far north regions began to develop almost explosively, the Lovelace Clinic, located on the southeast periphery of the city, found itself increasingly distant from the centers of the city's population growth. Either a way had to be found to induce patients to travel the extra distances to Gibson Boulevard for their everyday health-care needs, or the clinic had to go to them. The establishment of satellite clinics around the city ultimately proved to be one of the keys to the clinic's remarkable resurgence in the 1980s.

As early as 1967 the clinic's Board of Governors had discussed the idea of establishing some kind of extension of the clinic's services to newly developing areas in the city.[38] That discussion was stimulated by the board's consciousness of the city's demographic trends and their potential impact on the clinic's operations as well as by a growing concern and discussion of this issue by group practices elsewhere in the nation. The earliest experiments with branch or satellite clinics were not particularly successful, but several of the country's larger group practices continued to study the question. The decline of older, downtown areas, where most of the well established groups were located, and the rapid growth of suburban areas around the country, kept the issue high on their agendas.

In April 1970, a planning document drafted by a clinic administrator first projected construction of two Lovelace Clinic satellites, one in the far northeast heights and a second in Corrales.[39] By the end of that year, a rough consensus had been reached on the basic desirability of some kind of satellite effort, although agreement had not yet been reached on precisely where satellites should be placed, how they should be staffed and integrated within the overall institution, and how they might be financed.[40] In late 1971, the executive committee of the Board of Trustees approved the general idea and initiated concrete planning to identify financing options and the best possible branch sites.

38. Lovelace Clinic, Board of Governors, Minutes, 26 September 1967. A pioneering satellite—actually a kind of dispensary—had been established (appropriately) at the Albuquerque airport in 1965, not long before Randy Lovelace's death. That facility, limited to a kind of first-aid treatment and staffed by nursing personnel, was not economically viable and was closed shortly after Dr. Lovelace II's death. See ibid., 22 February 1966.

39. Dr. Jack Whenry, "A Five-Year-Plan for the Lovelace Clinic" (5 April 1970), copy in Lovelace Clinic, Board of Governors, Minutes, 21 April 1970.

40. Most often mentioned as likely sites for satellite development were the city's growing northwest section, especially the Rio Rancho-Corrales area, and the northeast heights; but that early discussion also included all quadrants of the city as well as towns of the surrounding region like Belen, Cochiti Lake, and Socorro. Lovelace Clinic, Board of Governors, Minutes, 30 June 1970, 22 September 1970, and passim.

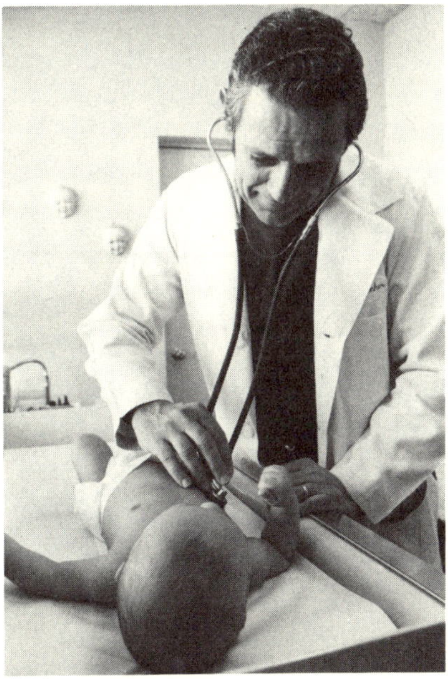

Dr. Paul Eicher was the much respected head of the Lovelace Clinic's pediatrics department from 1959 until his death in an airplane crash in 1977.

Funding was the main hindrance to rapid development of the satellite project, for this was precisely the time of acute financial woes within the Lovelace institution. External support played a major part in resolving the difficulty—specifically, Hill-Burton money from the federal government, plus a critically important grant of 400,000 dollars from the Robert Wood Johnson Foundation of Princeton, New Jersey. This East Coast foundation, active in many different spheres of the health-care field, was interested in the Lovelace effort as a part of its Community Hospital-Medical Staff Sponsored Group Practice Program, designed to encourage experimental projects in health-care delivery systems. When combined with institutional funds squeezed from the hard-pressed Lovelace Foundation budget, this external assistance permitted the program to get under way in May 1975, when a satellite clinic, staffed initially with three primary-care physicians (two internists and a pediatrician), opened in Rio Rancho on Albuquerque's northwest side. That pioneer venture was followed almost exactly two years later by the opening of a second satellite, on Juan Tabo in the city's

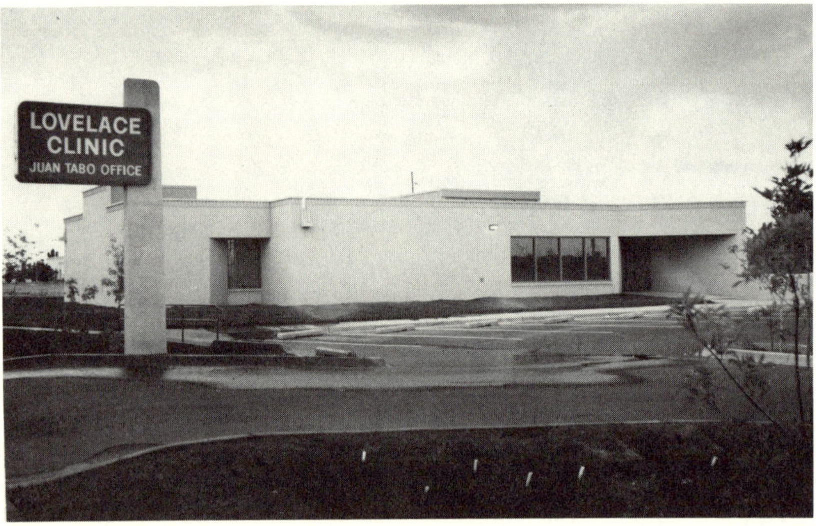

The Juan Tabo satellite was the second established in the Lovelace Clinic's highly successful satellite clinic program.

Northeast Heights region; and the attempt to expand beyond the confines of the Gibson Boulevard campus was in full operation.[41]

Throughout the first decade of the satellite experiment, many problems arose as the Lovelace innovators learned how best to manage and utilize the overall system; but it was also soon evident that the program was a resounding success. Immediately there were critical lessons to be learned regarding proper staffing of the satellite centers. The original impulse of the Lovelace leadership—to employ board-certified internists and pediatricians as the spearheads of the clinic's primary-care thrust, and thus as the backbone of the branch offices—quickly proved to be unsatisfactory. Within a relatively brief time, it was clear

41. The general details of the clinic's satellite program are readily available in the annual reports of the Lovelace Medical Center from 1973 to the present. The two original satellites were followed by a Corrales office (established in 1979, but merged with the Rio Rancho satellite in 1982); the Academy office (1982); San Pedro branch (1983); Rio Bravo and Tramway satellites (1984); a Santa Fe branch (1985); and a Carlisle Boulevard branch (1987). The total number of branches, with several offering extended service as urgent care centers, stood at eight in 1987.

that a large percentage of the patients who visited the satellites were seeking care for problems outside the normal sphere of an internist or pediatrician's practice. The stock in trade of the satellite physician included the sewing of a simple laceration, the provision of prenatal care, and the basic handling of a broken arm or a psychological problem, but these services required an expertise not all internists or pediatricians possessed. A crucial change in staffing philosophy at the Lovelace satellites came after the arrival of Dr. Ottensmeyer in 1976, with the institution committing itself wholeheartedly to the new and modern specialty called family practice. The skills and practice ethos of the new family-medicine practitioners fit well with the requirements of the satellite centers, and as the Lovelace satellite centers grew in numbers and patient volume, so too did the representation of family-medicine practitioners on the Lovelace staff. By 1986 no less than 34 of the 151 physicians on the staff were family-medicine specialists.[42]

The most obvious contribution of the satellite clinic program to the overall health and growth of the Lovelace institution lay in its impressive boost of patient volume. (See Table 7.) The total number of patient visits to the Lovelace Clinic had reached a plateau of around 160,000 to 170,000 annually in the sixties and seventies, but nearly tripled in the brief time from 1979 through 1985, reaching 460,000 visits in the latter year. While patients visits at the Gibson site rose by nearly two-thirds during that period, the bulk of the increase came through the satellites. Fewer than 6,000 total patient visits were registered during the first year of the Northwest Clinic's operation in 1975–76, but by 1985 the number of satellite visits soared to 200,000, a full 43 percent of the total for the Lovelace Clinic; and the Juan Tabo, Rio Rancho, and Rio Bravo branches had already been through a first round of physical expansion. The impact of the satellites on total patient volume also included a large number of patients first seen at one of the satellites, who were referred to the Gibson center for specialty care; this was,

42. On the importance of the shift to family medicine practitioners as a factor in making the satellite experiment work, see the Ottensmeyer interview, and Dr. Derick Pasternak, interview with the author, 21 April 1986 and passim.

Table 7 Patient Visits, Lovelace Clinic and Satellites, 1943–1985

Year	*Gibson Boulevard*	*Rio Rancho*	*Juan Tabo*	*Academy*	*San Pedro*	*Rio Bravo*	*Tramway*	*Santa Fe*	*Totals*
1943	45,074								45,074
1948	71,395								71,395
1960	152,333								152,333
1965	171,866								171,866
1970	184,470								184,470
1975									
1976									
1977	162,561	7,835	6,793*						177,189
1978	160,810	6,724	12,147						179,231
1979	151,994	9,096	17,739						178,829
1980									
1981	158,219	12,318	19,577						190,114
1982	171,995	16,030	22,939	3,427*					214,391
1983	199,236	21,073	34,013	18,056					272,378
1984	225,679	22,480	48,931	23,529	11,616	16,337			348,572
1985	260,923	29,194	51,972	40,133	17,573	29,778	17,821	11,490	458,884

*Partial year

of course, one of the main reasons for the satellites in the first place. Early studies conducted in 1979 indicated that at least one in every twenty patients seen at satellite clinics was referred to the Gibson site for specialist care,[43] and that figure almost surely underestimates the volume.

From 1973 to the late 1980s, the central importance of the satellite development program was reinforced by another successful experiment, the birth and growth at the Lovelace center of a pioneering health-maintenance organization (HMO).[44] Although prepaid medical plans have a history in the United States extending as far back as the 1920s, this alternative to traditional fee-for-service health-care organization first attracted considerable attention with the establishment of the Kaiser-Permanente health plan in California, initiated in the immediate post-World War Two era, and New York's Health

43. Lovelace Medical Foundation, *Annual Report*, 1979, p. 7.

44. As with the satellite program, the history of the Lovelace health maintenance organization is conveniently summarized in the Lovelace Medical Foundation annual reports from 1973 to the present.

Insurance Plan (HIP), inspired by New York City Mayor Fiorello La Guardia.[45] However, the influence of these health plans in the national medical marketplace remained limited; as late as 1971 there were no more than thirty health-maintenance organizations operating around the country. As the costs of health care skyrocketed in the late 1960s, the Nixon administration focused attention on what the president called "a new national health strategy" within which the HMO was a central component. To encourage the spread of the HMO concept of health delivery, the Nixon policymakers were able to push new legislation through Congress authorizing planning grants and loan guarantees for new HMO projects.[46] Within this highly supportive national context, the Lovelace leadership began to consider establishing a prepayment plan in the late 1960s.

The clinic's Board of Governors had first considered the prepaid medical-care concept, in what its minutes called "a rather heated discussion," in the fall of 1967.[47] California's Kaiser-Permanente system was the explicit model studied by the Lovelace authorities. The medical profession's intrinsic hostility toward what it regarded as a highly undesirable intrusion of economic considerations into the physician-patient relationship resulted in the Board of Governors' decision "that this was not a desirable feature for our community" and in a unanimous vote rejecting any further consideration of the issue.[48] However, two years later, when the entire subject was under vigorous discussion in professional journals and the national press and Congress was on the verge of passing legislation intended to aid financially widespread experimentation with health-maintenance organizations, Lovelace began to reconsider the matter. Dr. Kilgore, then chairman of the clinic's Board of Governors; H. Mikkel Kelly, chief administrator of Bataan Hospital and later

45. On the birth and development of prepaid health plans in this country, see Paul Starr, *The Social Transformation of American Medicine* (New York: Basic Books, 1982), esp. pp. 320–27.

46. For details of the HMO "revolution" of the seventies and the role of the federal government within it, see Joseph Falkson, *HMOs and the Politics of Health System Reform* (Chicago: American Hospital Association, 1980).

47. Lovelace Clinic, Board of Governors, Minutes, 10 October 1967.

48. Ibid.

vice president of administration of the Lovelace Center for the Health Sciences; and Joe Fulcher, the lawyer-manager responsible for administration of the Lovelace Foundation, constituted the leadership team which encouraged and guided the Lovelace institution's shift in position on the HMO question. They commissioned and directed feasibility studies, explored the opportunities for federal financial assistance, and began the essential in-house lobbying required to overcome the widespread suspicion of the new program. The national discussion of the question provided support for their local work by affording vitally needed information and exposure for the concept, thereby increasing the number of those willing to accept or at least to tolerate experimentation with an HMO.

Equally as important were two internal realities that predisposed the Lovelace institution toward a favorable attitude on the HMO question. In the first place, a moderately sized health plan promised to provide a vitally needed capital infusion for the financially troubled institution. All of the planning documents of the early seventies emphasized the potential utility of "up front cash" in helping the clinic to improve its financial position.[49] Second, the Lovelace leadership was convinced that the prepaid health care concept was just another manifestation of the organizational principle, one of the guiding precepts of group practices such as the Lovelace Clinic. Just as group practice represented a logical, efficient, and progressive approach to the practice of medicine, and the merger of the three Lovelace health-care institutions then underway on the Lovelace campus heralded a step toward more effective coordination and management of interrelated health enterprises, so too did provision of a well-managed prepaid health plan constitute another important step toward the integrated health-care delivery system of the future.

Although there was much activity devoted to steering the Lovelace Clinic toward trial of an HMO—Dr. Kilgore thought it clearly "the wave of the future"—there remained a great deal

49. See, for example, Dr. Jack L. Whenry, "Establishing a Group Practice Pre-Payment Plan," memorandum to Board of Governors, 19 May 1970.

of residual suspicion and even hostility. For example, Medical Director Mowry was opposed to an HMO at Lovelace and determined that if it had to become a reality, he would see to it that it affected the actual practice of medicine at the center as little as possible.[50] Certification of patient membership in the health plan was to be strictly a business office matter and of no concern to the practicing physician. The collapse of this first Lovelace venture into the HMO business was almost preordained by the failure to acknowledge that patient-members of a health plan emphatically demand much greater quantities of health care and the related failure to establish anything like a "gatekeeper" to appraise the types and dimensions of health care appropriate in any particular case. Nevertheless, in 1971 and 1972, with the assistance of a federal-government planning grant, Lovelace began its preparations for establishing an HMO, the first in New Mexico and in the entire region from Dallas-Fort Worth to Phoenix. The intention was to start with a small program, and then, after shaking the flaws from the system through two or three years of operation, to expand the operation decisively, perhaps to include as many as thirty thousand members. The pace of development would be controlled by experience with the capitation system itself and by the ease of accommodation within the clinic to the new operation.

The Lovelace-Bataan Health Program, originally called Mediguard, began to operate in January 1973, and within two years it was almost moribund, a grand experiment which had proved to be a grave disappointment to its sponsoring institution. A major part of its difficulties arose from the nature of the clientele selected for service under the new health plan. Its initial marketing efforts in late 1972 and early 1973 were aimed at the scientists and technicians of Albuquerque's Sandia National Laboratories and the professionals and other employees of the city's University of New Mexico; and both of these groups became intolerably high users of medical services. (During that

50. A colleague who admired Dr. Mowry's zealous dedication to quality medical care, as he saw it, summarized the situation succinctly: "While Don Kilgore thought it [an HMO] the wave of the future, Frank Mowry thought it the spawn of the devil." Private communication.

early period, only the employees of the City of Albuquerque proved to be an economically manageable service group.) In the complete absence of any kind of control over the services rendered, the roughly five thousand members of the Lovelace health plan imposed a large-scale fiscal drain on the institution's resources, rather than providing the financial boost which had been anticipated. Dropping both the laboratory and the university groups provided a measure of financial relief, but by the fall of 1975 membership in the plan had shrunk to a little more than three thousand members; and there was growing sentiment that Lovelace should simply terminate the entire effort.[51] That was certainly the position of Medical Director Mowry as well as others within the Lovelace center; but Dr. Kilgore continued to insist that, even though it obviously needed reformation, Lovelace's best interests would be served by staying with the health plan.[52] The pressure to junk the whole enterprise was successfully resisted, but the commitment of the institution to its HMO remained equivocal.

During the three or four years that followed, a time when the energies of the new Ottensmeyer administration were focused on rebuilding the medical staff and coping with the serious financial problems of the institution, the expansion of the system distinctly took second place to the internal reorganization and adjustments necessary to make it work profitably. (It was also recognized that the future of the prepayment plan was intimately linked to the development of the infrastructure to support it; in particular, a strong primary-care capability within the institution and the satellite clinics that would make Lovelace readily accessible to its potential HMO customers.) One major internal adjustment within the HMO was already in motion when Dr. Ottensmeyer arrived. In the summer of 1976, experimentation began with "a new utilization control program . . . involving a Primary Care Physician,"[53] which was

51. Lovelace Clinic, Board of Governors, Minutes, 7 October 1975; Lovelace-Bataan Medical Center, *Annual Report*, 1975, p. 18.

52. As already mentioned, this difference of opinion over the HMO was the major substantive issue in the clash between the two.

53. Lovelace Center for the Health Sciences, *Annual Report*, 1976, p. 10.

a key change in determining the future success of the plan. This change was accompanied by intensified efforts to win the medical staff's cooperation and unqualified support for the HMO enterprise, as well as by managerial and administrative changes designed to effect tighter control over expenditures and to develop marketing strategies for an eventual expansion of the program.[54]

A firm institutional commitment to the health plan was formally made in 1977, and in 1979 a number of developments evolved from that commitment. An experienced, strong administrator, William H. Townsend, was hired at the beginning of that year as executive director of the health plan, and charged with presiding over its expansion. The decision was made to seek federal qualification of the Lovelace HMO, in order to open up access to additional federal assistance—in exchange for an open-membership policy within the plan. To reflect a new start, the name of the operation was changed to the more straightforward Lovelace Health Plan. In 1980, federal assistance made it possible to hire a finance manager and a marketing director as well as to purchase sophisticated computer equipment that would aid in controlling the operation.

More important, however, than these financial and administrative preparations was the crucial, and sometimes difficult, conversion of the medical staff to the realization that skillful, tasteful marketing was indispensable to the success of an aggressive HMO. Physicians educated in the postwar era were still reared in the tradition that any form of marketing or promotion was "advertising" in the most pejorative sense of the word and to be shunned as beneath the dignity of the profession. In the 1970s, however, some among them began to realize that, as medicine became increasingly competitive and more closely integrated within the corporate structure of the American business world, then some form of marketing was inevitable. During the late 1970s and early 1980s, the leaders of the Lovelace Clinic undertook the somewhat unpopular job of educating their colleagues to the realities of the changing world

54. Lovelace Center for the Health Sciences, Medical Staff, Minutes, 11 July 1977.

of health care and eventually won their support for a strong, forthright marketing program which began in 1982. The charge of "advertizing" was quickly raised, but the AMA's 1976 liberalization of its position on the advertising question had already cut the ground from under the feet of the Lovelace critics, and Dr. Ottensmeyer's spirited defense of the Lovelace position before the Bernalillo County Medical Association effectively drove the opposition underground. The firm and unapologetic acceptance of marketing by the Lovelace staff was a crucial factor in the success of the Lovelace Health Plan, and it was another mark of Lovelace's leadership within the profession at large.

With everything in place and careful plans formulated the big expansion of the Lovelace Health Plan began in 1981. Table 8 plots its remarkable growth over the following few years. From merely 3,600 members in 1980, the plan shot to more than 56,000 in 1985, a more than fifteenfold increase; and in doing so, it became a centrally important element in the overall Lovelace operations. Much of the remarkably rapid growth in patient visits to the clinic, so evident in Table 7, is directly attributable to the growth of the HMO; and by mid-1986 the plan accounted for 54 percent of the total business of the clinic. The extraordinary pace of the plan's growth was determined by several factors: the maturation of the satellite program and that of the primary-care staffing strategy; the absence of HMO competition locally during the critical early part of the eighties;[55] the hard-earned reputation of the clinic for excellence and leadership in clinical medicine; and the well-conceived and orchestrated marketing campaign. As the decade unfolded, the Lovelace Health Plan blossomed as one of the most important spheres of the entire Lovelace complex. Indeed, as early as the middle of the decade, there was talk on the Lovelace campus and among the institution's trustees of the health plan as "the tail wagging the dog."[56] There was certainly no question that the venture had played a vital role in the powerful resurgence of the Lovelace center during the eighties—from about 8 percent

55. Presbyterian and St. Joseph hospitals backed a locally organized and controlled HMO called Mastercare in the late seventies, but the experiment was halted in 1980.

56. Private communication.

Table 8 Lovelace Health Plan (HMO) Membership, 1973–1986

Year	*Membership*
1973	2,200
1974	6,000
1975	
1976	3,500
1977	
1978	
1979	
1980	3,600
1981	5,900
1982	12,900
1983	24,900
1984	41,400
1985	56,000
1986	69,800

of the area's clinical practice in 1976, Lovelace rose to approximately 20 percent in 1985—and that the institution had established itself as both a regional and national leader in the reshaping of the structure of the American health-care delivery system near the end of the twentieth century.

Although the development of the clinic absorbed much of the Lovelace leadership's time and energies during the period from 1965 to the mid-1980s, medical research continued to enjoy special prestige and emphasis. Expansion of the foundation's research program continued, even though there was a marked shift of focus as the earlier emphasis on aviation-aerospace medicine waned and its place of primacy was taken by a large-scale program of inhalation toxicology research. To a considerable degree, progress was attributable to the continuity in leadership and vision afforded through Randy Lovelace's close friend and colleague, Dr. Sam White. Within days of the airplane crash that took Randy's life, Dr. White was selected as his successor as president of the Lovelace Foundation, and for another decade—until his resignation in 1974, to accept the presidency of the Oklahoma Medical Research Foundation—

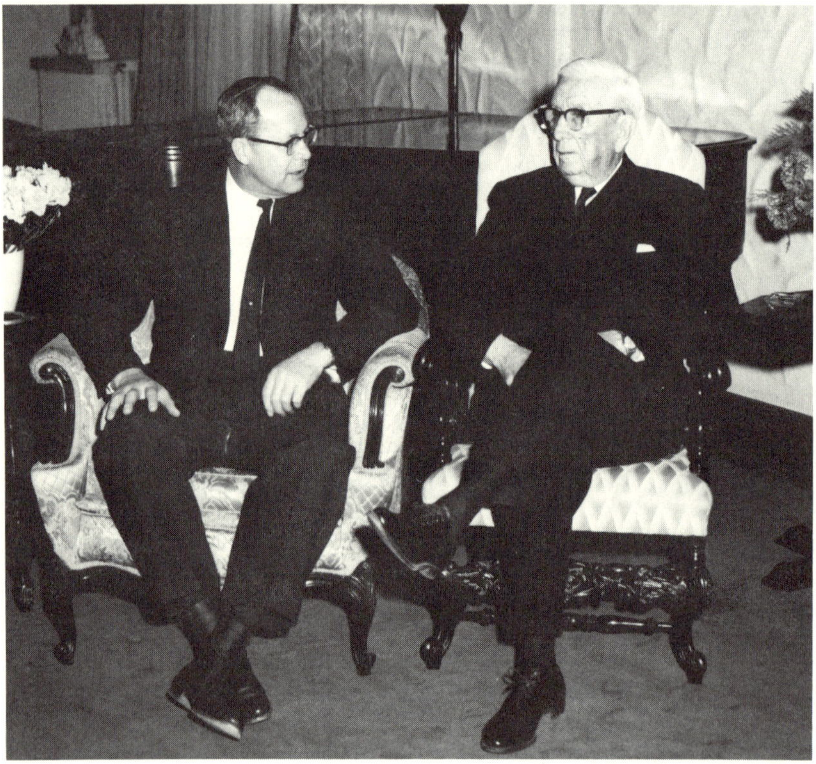

Dr. Sam White, left, was chosen to succeed Randy Lovelace as President of the Lovelace Foundation. He is shown in this late 1965 photograph, just days after the death of Randy Lovelace, with the aged "Uncle Doc" Lovelace.

Sam White directed the research program of the Lovelace scientific team. In the fifties, he had been the father of the foundation's blast and shock biology project, the research work that had been so central to the establishment of the Albuquerque center's reputation and the building of its staff. Throughout the 1960s, he guided the early years of the second major research effort, which within a startlingly brief period of time, developed into a multimillion-dollar enterprise with a large interdisciplinary staff that rapidly earned worldwide distinction in the field of inhalation toxicology research. In addition, the Lovelace Foundation sponsored a broad array of clinical research projects, reaffirming the tradition of versatility and creativity that had distinguished its earlier years.

The special interest in inhalation toxicology at the Lovelace center grew from several sources—Dr. White's wartime studies of aerosols for the U.S. Navy and Ulrich Luft's work in pulmonary physiology foremost among them. That interest, combined with the success of the blast biology investigations, which had firmly established the scientific credibility and capability of the Lovelace researchers, made the Lovelace center an attractive candidate in the 1950s when the U.S. Atomic Energy Commission began to seek scientific assistance with some of its radiation studies. In the mid-1950s the government agency sponsored programs at various laboratories around the nation to study the potential health effects of radiation, including radionuclides that might be inhaled and deposited within the body. The federal agency, of course, was particularly concerned with radionuclide toxicity problems that might be encountered in the development, manufacture, testing, and possible use of nuclear weapons, and then, somewhat later, with those associated with the generation of power in the rapidly expanding nuclear power industry. Lovelace became involved in this work in the summer of 1959, when the AEC's Division of Biology and Medicine, the original sponsor of Lovelace's blast and shock biology program, approached Dr. White, the director of research, to inquire about the possible interest of the Albuquerque institution in pursuing research focused on inhaled fission product radionuclides.[57] Dr. White formulated a basic proposal which was submitted to the federal authorities in January 1960, and by June of that year approval of his plans had been received.

The first few years of the Lovelace program were devoted essentially to building the specialized staff needed for the new program, especially in the fields of aerosol physics, radiobiology, and animal care and management, and in the construction of special facilities to house the work. (Early work was carried

57. For a good survey history of the Lovelace work in inhalation toxicology, see Roger O. McClellan, "Twenty-five Years of Lovelace Research in Inhalation Toxicology," in *From Sundagger to Space Exploration: Significant Scientific Contributions to Science and Technology in New Mexico*, special issue of *New Mexico Journal of Science* 26 (1986):330–45. See also the Inhalation Toxicology Research Institute file in the Lovelace Medical Center archives and Dr. Roger O. McClellan, interview with the author, Albuquerque, 1 August 1985.

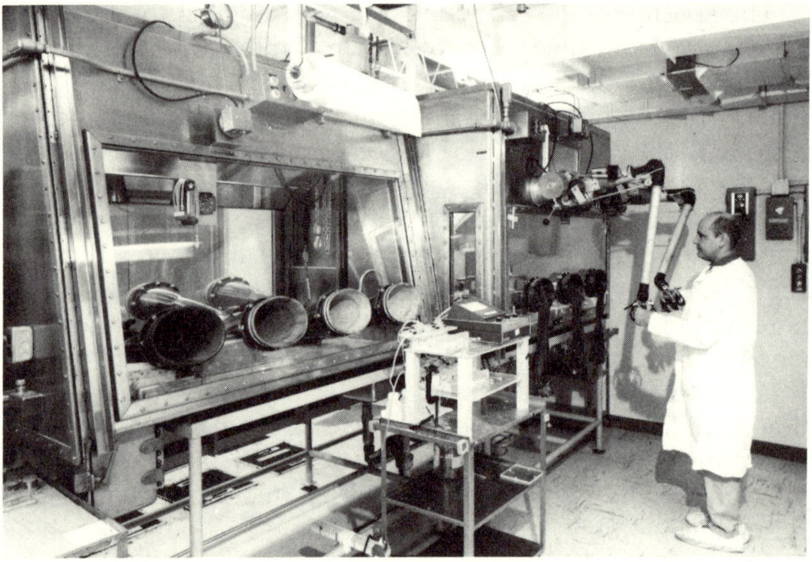

Remote handling equipment for working with high levels of radioactivity is a part of the specialized apparatus used in research on the toxicology of inhaled radionuclides.

out in the foundation headquarters buildings on Gibson Boulevard and at the Lovelace blast site on Sandia Base, but construction of permanent facilities adjacent to the blast and shock biology complex on south Sandia Base, whose name was later changed to Kirtland Air Force Base, quickly followed.) The original plans for the Lovelace program called for its studies to focus on several animal species—in particular, Beagle dogs, guinea pigs, rats, and mice which would be exposed for experimental purposes to radioactive aerosols. The work began with efforts directed toward the development of techniques for producing and characterizing aerosols that could be used to expose the test animals in a highly reproducible fashion. Key features of the exposure systems were the development of both large-animal and small-animal plethysmographs to measure the respiratory activity of animals during exposure and techniques for working with highly radioactive materials. New Departments of Aerosol Physics and Radiobiology were established and the already existing staffs of the foundation's Departments of Biochemistry, Microbiology, and Pathology were expanded to provide the sophisticated biomedical support required in evaluating the clinical effects of inhaled radioactive materials.

The inhalation toxicology program grew swiftly, and within five years it employed the equivalent of twenty-four full-time scientific and engineering professionals as well as a corps of specially trained technical and support personnel. Its budget climbed in that same period to over 1.7 million dollars, 53 percent of the total foundation budget, and its physical facilities grew remarkably. The initial building devoted to the program was opened on the air force base site in 1963, and included more than 80,000 square feet of space. The first scholarly papers produced by the new research team appeared in 1962. In the formative years of the program's development, Dr. White directed its work, but his elevation to the foundation's presidency in late 1965 required him to turn over research direction to someone else. An experienced and highly effective scientist-manager was found in Dr. Roger O. McClellan, who joined the Lovelace staff as director of the Fission Product Inhalation Program in September 1966.[58] Dr. McClellan, a doctor of veterinary medicine with ten years' experience in AEC-sponsored radiation effects work, proved to be a brilliant success in the job. Under his direction, the Lovelace toxicology program grew from its strong foundations to international stature.

Part of Dr. McClellan's special charge was to broaden the program from its originally exclusive focus on the radionuclides produced in the fission process. That expansion of the program's scope began in the late sixties, when the inhalation toxicity of plutonium and other transuranic radionuclides produced in plutonium recycle reactors came under study; but it was the 1970s that witnessed an important qualitative change in the program's operations. To their ongoing work focused on the dangers of inhaling fission products, in the seventies the Lovelace researchers added new investigations involving a broad array of chemical toxicants. Much of the impetus for that shift

58. Twenty years later, as this is written, Dr. McClellan remained head of the inhalation toxicology work.

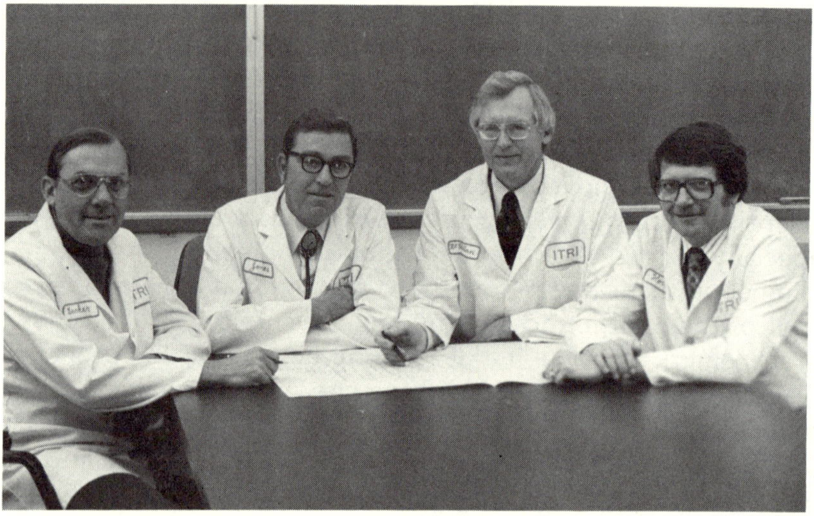

Leaders of the Inhalation Toxicology Research Institute posed for this 1980 photograph. Left to right: Dr. Bruce B. Boecker, assistant director; Dr. Robert K. Jones, associate director; Dr. Roger O. McClellan, director; and Dr. Charles H. Hobbs, assistant director.

came from the environmentalism of the 1970s, as society grew increasingly concerned about the health hazards associated with the fouling of the atmosphere; but much came from the internal logic of the Lovelace work itself. It was natural to transfer the expertise and techniques gleaned in the study of the radionuclides to other potentially dangerous substances inhaled by people in their everyday world, and federal government funding encouraged the Lovelace scientists to broaden their studies. The expanded program drew support from the National Institutes of Health, the U.S. Food and Drug Administration, and the Consumer Product Safety Commission to fund investigation of the toxicity of aerosolized consumer products; and the Department of Energy provided money to initiate studies on the toxicity of diesel exhaust emissions, man-made insulating fibers, and various heat transfer fluids used in solar energy applications. Other chemical toxicants were added to the growing list of substances under investigation as the diversification process intensified, and in 1973 the name of the Fission Product

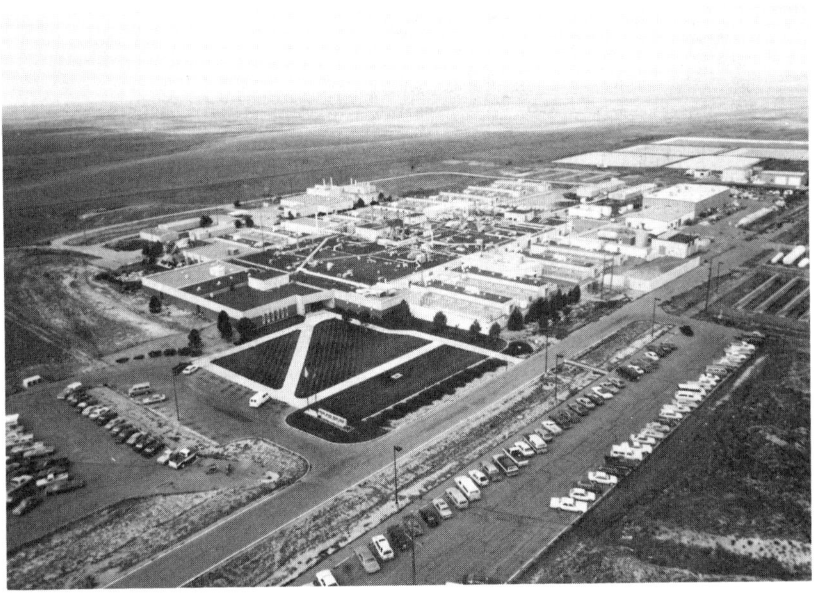

An aerial view of the Inhalation Toxicology Research Institute facility, around 1985.

Inhalation Program was changed to the Inhalation Toxicology Research Institute (ITRI) to reflect the broader purview of its work. By 1980 over half the research program of ITRI involved non-nuclear studies, with 54 percent of its 11.5 million dollar budget (1984) devoted to chemical toxicology investigation and another 6 percent to other, non-nuclear work.

As the fission product work matured and other fields of study opened up, the physical facilities of the ITRI grew to include more than 220 thousand square feet of space with equipment valued at approximately 33 million dollars. The staff expanded to fifty professionals with doctoral degrees plus another 190 support personnel—technicians, animal care specialists, clerical and plant personnel—and the output of scholarly papers by the institution's researchers grew to eighty to one hundred per year in the mid-eighties. The institute also played a major role in the overall educational work of the Lovelace center, providing a broad range of educational activities. For example, a student research program initiated in 1967 included

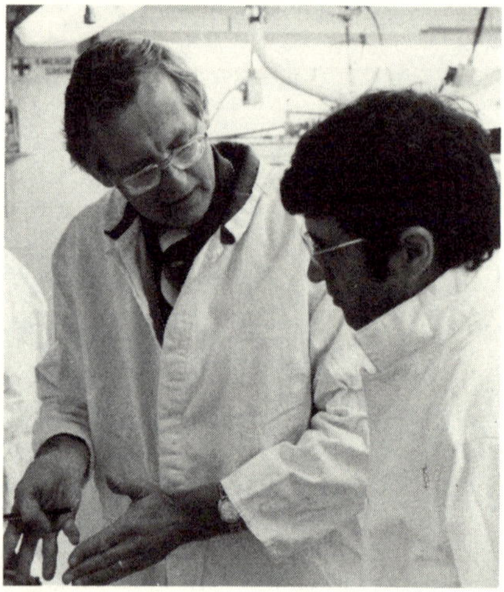

Dr. Roger McClellan, director of the Inhalation Toxicology Research Institute, describes a project to Senator Harrison "Jack" Schmitt. Schmitt, the astronaut-geologist who was the last man to walk on the moon, joined the Lovelace Foundation's Board of Trustees in 1985 and chaired its research committee.

more than 500 students from fifty schools in more than twenty states during the first two decades of its existence. Graduate students at both master's and doctoral degree level regularly conducted thesis and dissertation research at the institute, and ten to twelve postdoctoral fellows per year pursued their studies at the Lovelace facility. Administratively the Inhalation Toxicology Research Institute was treated as a separate operating division of the Lovelace Foundation until 1975 when the Lovelace Biomedical and Environmental Research Institute (LBERI) was created as a nonprofit subsidiary of the Lovelace Foundation for the sole purpose of operating the toxicology research institute. Though physically and administratively removed somewhat from the other elements of the Lovelace medical complex, it remained a critical part of the Lovelace family of health care institutions and brought international attention to the Albuquerque medical center.

The inhalation toxicology research program overshadowed other research work at the Lovelace center—with the solitary exception of the physiology program directed by Dr. Luft—until the 1980s when strong, new leadership rejuvenated the Foundation's constricted clinical research efforts. While direction of the inhalation toxicology work was highly centralized in the capable hands of Dr. McClellan and tightly focused in

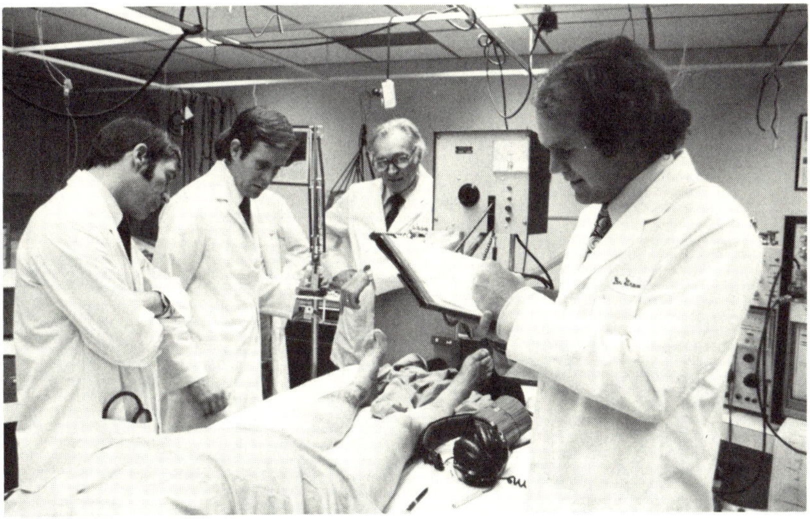

Foundation scientist-researcher Dr. Richard E. "Dick" Greene demonstrates new equipment and techniques to surgeons (left to right) Dr. James Larkin, Dr. Earl Badger, and Dr. Jack McCarthy.

its scope of operations and objectives, the clinical research efforts carried out by the Lovelace researchers were much less closely coordinated and integrated. The orienting focus of aviation-aerospace medicine diminished markedly, especially after the departure of Dr. White in 1974, and the entire clinical research program suffered gravely from lack of financial support. With the exception of Dr. Luft's pulmonary physiology studies, supported by NASA grants, the clinical research operations of the Foundation were largely dependent on Board of Trustees funds—in-house money—and those funds were severely restricted in the late sixties and seventies. An administrative reorganization in 1976 made a major difference in the fortunes of the clinical research efforts of the Foundation. In that year all the Gibson-site research work was organized into a new Clinical Research Division and placed under central leadership. The appointment to that post in 1978 of Dr. Waneta Tuttle, a locally trained physiologist-student of Dr. Luft, was the starting point for an impressive revival of Lovelace's clinical research efforts in the 1980s.

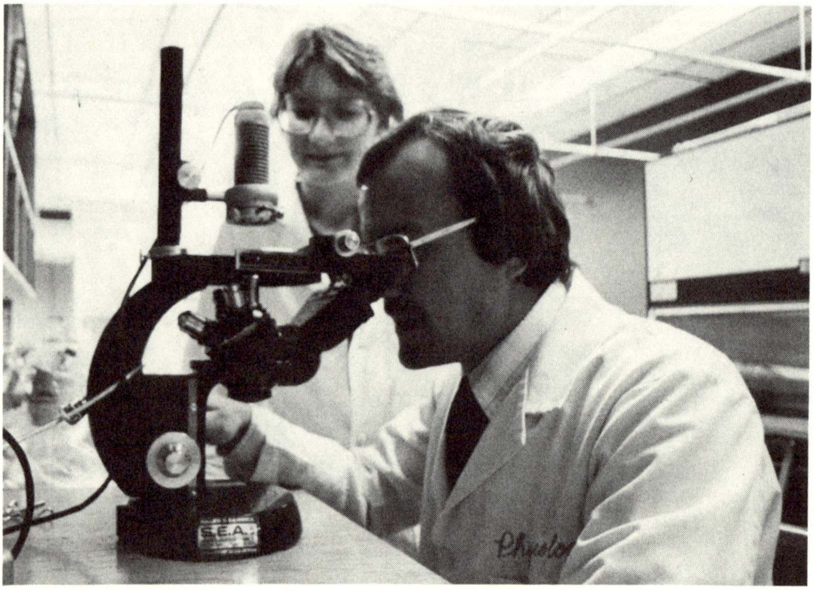

Foundation rheumatologist Dr. Robert Searles at work, assisted by lab specialist Karla Ojanen.

Dr. Tuttle began her tenure in office by presiding over a major planning study in 1979 designed to re-evaluate the mission, objectives, and possibilities of the Clinical Research Division as well as its relationships within the overall Lovelace complex. From that process (and the new energy injected into the division) came a new program for the 1980s focused around cell biology and biomedical engineering and committed to the aggressive pursuit of outside grant funding to undergird the entire endeavor. The results were quick and impressive. From a 400 thousand dollar level of funding for the entire division in 1980, revenues swelled to approximately 2.2 million dollars within a five year span, most of the increase achieved through outside support. Studies within the Division involved non-invasive blood flow investigations, particularly intracardiac flow studies and peripheral vascular blood flow work using Doppler echocardiography; development of new, sophisticated instrumentation to carry out those studies, especially new instruments involving pulsed Doppler ultrasound techniques; the investigation of connective tissue disease, especially arthritis

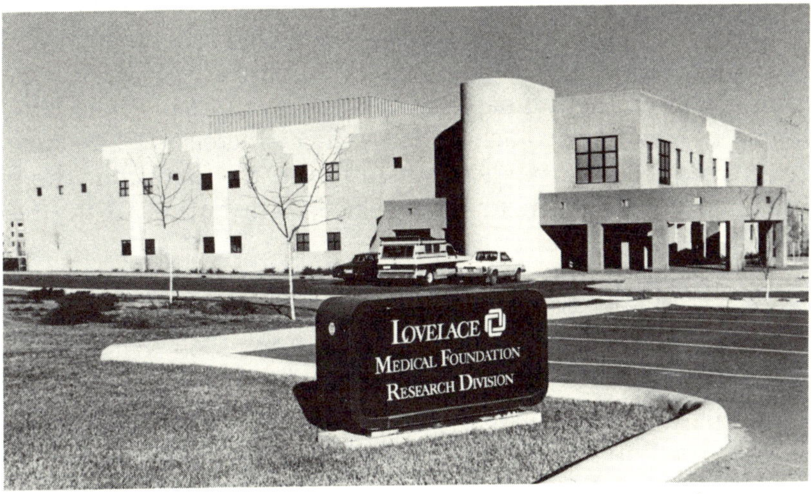

The new Lovelace Medical Foundation Research building, opened in 1984.

(the Division's Dr. Robert Searles in 1980 got a three-year Clinical Investigator Award from the National Institute of Arthritis, Metabolism, and Digestive Disease); and a broad range of other studies, many with immediate clinical applications. Toward the end of the eighties, the efforts of the Division concentrated on work with technology focuses in the areas of nuclear magnetic resonance, including its immunodiagnostic applications; acoustic imaging and flowmetry; markers for DNA damage and repair; and immunodiagnostics in general. In addition, the Division developed special programs in health services research and was successful in late 1984 in winning a three-year, 36 million dollar federal contract to study the effects, if any, of Agent Orange exposure on Vietnam veterans. This surge of new energy and pioneering of new fields of activity by the Clinical Research Division was crowned symbolically with the opening of a new, thirty-one thousand square foot Research Division building on the southeastern edge of the Gibson campus, a physical symbol of Lovelace's enduring commitment to excellence in clinical research.

Progress within the medical education component of the Lovelace Foundation's overall mission was less dynamic in the seventies and eighties, but the Foundation nonetheless remained deeply involved in medical education at several different levels. Its educational programs had grown moderately prior to 1965, even though its efforts and ambitions had been constrained seriously by financial limits. After 1964 the new University of New Mexico School of Medicine increasingly became the central focus of medical education in the state, but there remained ample room for a Lovelace contribution to the region's medical educational needs.

Lovelace continued, for example, its involvement in graduate medical education, assisting in the training of nearly two hundred residents during the period from 1965 to the mid-eighties. In the late sixties, the five residency programs it had established over the preceding decade—in general medicine, radiology, pathology, general surgery, and pediatrics—were integrated fully with those established at the new medical school, but Lovelace continued to fund 15 residents and fellows in programs directed by UNM authorities. It also provided clerkships and other forms of clinical instruction for third and fourth year medical students from the local school, with fifty to eighty students per year receiving at least a part of their clinical instruction at Lovelace. Nursing students, too, from local nursing schools rotated through the Lovelace hospital.

The relationship with the university was a difficult one. Many on the Lovelace campus felt the connection was decidedly one way, the school of medicine taking far more than it gave.[59] Consistently throughout the seventies and eighties, Lovelace spent considerable sums of money on its graduate and undergraduate education programs—actual cash outlay in fiscal year 1975–76 was roughly 300 thousand dollars, *not* counting physician time spent teaching (estimated at another 150 thousand dollars)—and in return got some house officer service at its hospital, the prestige (and recruiting advantage) associated with status as a teaching hospital, and some academic appointments. However, the feeling persisted that its assistance to the school of medicine was not sufficiently recognized and appreciated, and in 1977, a time of acute financial stringency

59. Lovelace Medical Center, Medical Staff, Minutes, 26 October 1977 and private communications.

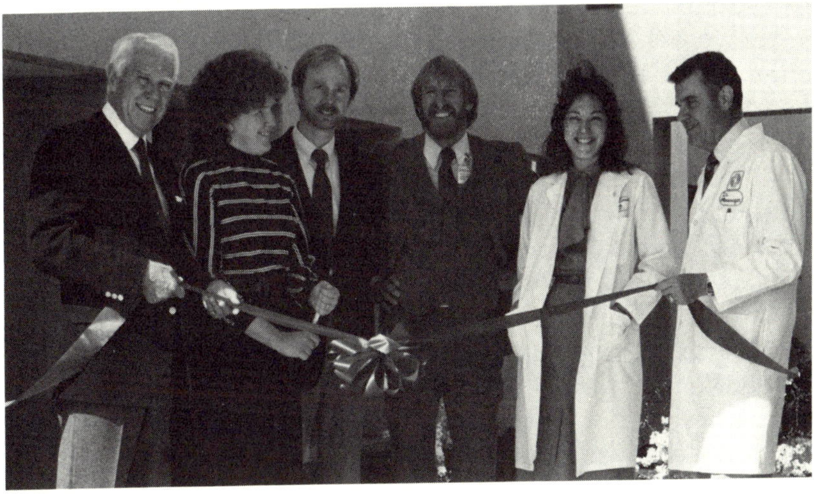

Celebrants at the opening of the new Lovelace Medical Foundation Research building. Left to right: Horace McKay, vice-chairman of the foundation's Board of Trustees; Dr. Waneta Tuttle, vice-president of the foundation and its chief operating officer; Jerry Davis, director of the foundation's Bioengineering Research division; Dr. Ken Ley, director of Biomedical Research for the foundation; Dr. Teresa Coons, staff scientist; and Dr. David J. Ottensmeyer, president and chief executive officer of the Lovelace Medical Center at the time of the 1984 opening.

within the organization, Lovelace's commitment to cooperation within the university's program was temporarily cut back. For its part, the medical school had the delicate political task of walking a narrow line between the large, well-organized group practice-foundation, whose assistance it properly desired and needed within its educational mission, and the sophisticated, politically alert and powerful private practice community of Albuquerque, which was always wary of the influence of the Lovelace center within the new medical school. For these reasons, full integration and coordination of the educational work of the Lovelace institution and that of the university remained elusive, a challenge to the future.[60]

60. For a thoughtful summary of the relationship between the two institutions and a projection of how things could be improved, see Dr. Clayton S. White to Dr. Lawrence H. Wilkinson [regent of the University of New Mexico], 14 September 1970, a letter held in the Lovelace Medical Center archives.

Though the residencies and medical student teaching programs were the most demanding and costly components of the foundation's educational work, it contributed at other levels of the spectrum as well. Intramural programs for medical staff and other employees included a variety of continuing education opportunities for physicians—departmental conferences and colloquia, formal grand rounds, visiting professor-lecturer seminars, and the like—continuing education programs, including formal course work for nurses and technical personnel, and a constantly broadening range of non-medical courses—Spanish for Medical Personnel, management courses like Time Management, Preventive Labor Relations, and others—for all within the medical center. Patient education programs plus fifty continuing education seminars for practicing physicians eager to refurbish or expand their knowledge fleshed out the range of educational efforts at the Lovelace campus. Coordination of the overall program and responsibility for it rested in the hands of the foundation's Director of Medical Education, a position held from 1973 by Dr. Martin J. Conway, an endocrinologist who had joined the Clinic in 1968. Much of the strength and success of the Lovelace educational effort in the seventies and eighties was derived from the stability of the program under Dr. Conway and from his personal commitment to the educational mission of the institution.[61] Patients, practicing physicians around the state, employees and staff of the Lovelace institution, undergraduate medical students, and graduate physicians together constituted the broad clientele served by the Lovelace educational effort, a commitment pursued at considerable institutional effort and cost over the years.

The pioneering tradition that has so decisively marked the history of the Lovelace medical center since Uncle Doc Lovelace's 1906 pioneering in Sunnyside, New Mexico, was rein-

61. Dr. Conway's dedication to medical education was reflected in his selection by students of the University of New Mexico School of Medicine to receive the school's Khatali Award in 1975, an award given to a faculty member "for unswerving dedication to his patients and students." Conway was the first non-regular faculty member to be given the distinction.

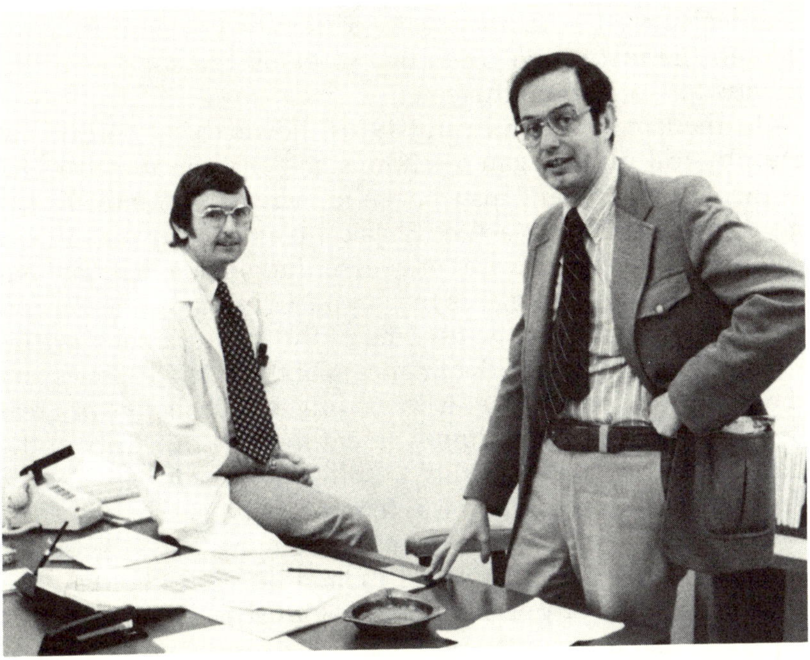

Leaders of the Lovelace Foundation educational effort. Left, Dr. Martin Conway, director of medical education, 1973 to the present, and, right, Dr. Derick Pasternak, associate director of medical education, 1975–1980. (In 1986 Dr. Pasternak became president and chief executive officer of the Lovelace Medical Center.)

forced in the mid-1980s when Lovelace linked its future with that of one of the corporate giants of the late twentieth-century American health scene. One of the major weaknesses of the Albuquerque institution in the sixties and seventies had been its chronic shortage of capital. Through the first two decades of the existence of the Lovelace Foundation, capital for building purposes or for the purchase of major equipment had been raised on an ad hoc basis by appealing to the generosity of the institution's friends and supporters. That policy had worked well enough through the late forties and fifties, but was dangerously dependent on the energies and contacts of one individual. It also meant that any kind of systematic planning and development was difficult. That approach to capital accumulation collapsed with the death of Randy Lovelace in 1965, though the institution continued to enjoy the support of his friends for some time thereafter.

In the late 1960s and early 1970s, however, as portions of the physical plant began to show signs of wear and tear and as medical equipment costs began to increase enormously, the need for capital grew acute. Physical plant improvement and equipment updating were, of course, high priority items, but so, too, were such things as the support of staff expansion and salary improvements; the funding of the institutional reorganization then underway; the financing of the satellite clinics and the HMO; and much else. It was a financial challenge of great urgency, and upon its solution rested the basic integrity of the Lovelace center and its ability to fulfill its mission.

The short-term solution was to resort to the use of industrial revenue bonds to address some of the more pressing capital needs. In 1978, for example, 11 million dollars in bonds were sold through the City of Albuquerque Industrial Revenue Bonds program, and the money used to finance a badly needed major remodeling program and the purchase of overdue new equipment. The success of that first bond issue resulted in a second in 1981—with the first two bond issues together producing around 22 million dollars for the institution's use—and a third, smaller one in 1983. Those funds were vital in purchasing "catch-up" equipment, in renovation and remodeling work, and in financing part of the satellite clinic program, but none of that capital was used in addressing the increasingly worrisome problem of the aging of Bataan Hospital. At the start of the 1980s, Bataan Hospital, for all its proud heritage, was in fact a thirty-year-old institution. Built to the standards of the 1940s and early 1950s, it was costly to operate, requiring 4.2 employees per patient while the typical modern hospital got along with 3.2, and beginning to show its age physically. It was a difficult and costly plant to modify as well, for every remodeling project exposed the Lovelace planners to the requirement of having to meet the more demanding building, fire, and safety codes of the seventies and eighties.[62]

62. Ottensmeyer, interview, 23 August 1985.

There were two broad alternatives for solving the hospital problem. First of all, there was the option of trying to keep ahead of the decay of the hospital plant by a policy of extensive remodeling and repair, a kind of "patch up" and preventive maintenance strategy. That approach was unappealing for many because it was essentially a "bandaid" solution to a fundamental problem which was not going to disappear, but rather to worsen with time. Further, planning studies done in the early eighties indicated the costs of that approach would probably be too much for the institution to bear.[63] The other alternative was to replace the hospital with an entirely new structure, a relatively quick and decisive solution to the difficulty, but one estimated to cost at least 40 to 45 million dollars. The Lovelace Foundation did not have such capital available to it, nor was it easy to see where it might be secured. It was, then, the need to replace its hospital which opened the Lovelace institution in the early eighties to the search for a partner.

In the early 1980s, when Lovelace began to consider the necessity for abandoning its traditional "stand-alone" policy, there was a range of possibilities open to it. One option involved the formation of a partnership locally with Southwest Community Health Services, the parent organization of Albuquerque's Presbyterian Hospital. There was much to commend the idea of merging these two leaders of the local health care market. The two institutions were roughly equal in size and strength;[64] each had a proud, distinctive tradition of service to the Albuquerque and New Mexico communities of their birth and growth; and each had a strong reputation for excellence and innovation in health care delivery. The combination of their resources would produce an institution of sufficient size and strength to compete effectively in the increasingly tough and demanding health-care delivery environment of the end of the century. In addition, there was a certain natural complementarity of the two institutions which seemed to suggest a special logic to their combination: Presbyterian's strength lay in its

63. Lovelace Medical Foundation, Board of Trustees, Annual Meeting, 1985, Minutes, p. E-20.

64. Total assets of Presbyterian Hospital in 1977 were estimated at 36.2 million dollars and those of Lovelace-Bataan Medical Center at 22.2 million dollars.

hospital system—it had the modern beds and a proven hospital administration system to manage them—and Lovelace had the organized medical staff and, with its booming HMO, the patients.[65]

Serious talks between the two institutions regarding their possible combination began in late 1976 with discussions climaxing early the next year.[66] Broad areas of agreement were quickly developed in the course of the talks, with both sides obviously very much interested in their possible combination, but the whole initiative shattered on the resistance of the "downtown docs" on whom Presbyterian Hospital Center relied for support of its hospitals. Faced with the anxiety and hostility of influential segments of the private practice community, where anti-Lovelace sentiment had historically been strong and only recently fanned to new intensity by the exodus of so many erstwhile Lovelace staffers out into the community, the Presbyterian authorities decided to suspend negotiations for a time, and the wary courtship between the two sides was in essence broken off.[67] Almost six years later, when Lovelace began to grapple seriously with the problem of replacing its hospital, new proposals were made for linkage of the two native institutions and a new series of discussions ensued. Once again the talks failed to bear fruit, even though they did reach the stage of a formal set of proposals suggesting a merger of the two institutions.[68]

In 1983, while the negotiations with Presbyterian Hospital unfolded, Lovelace was first approached by national concerns interested in a possible association with the Albuquerque in-

65. Interviews with Dr. Ottensmeyer and Robert O. Anderson and the files of the Lovelace Clinic's Board of Governors and Medical Staff. See, for example, Lovelace Clinic, Medical Staff, Minutes, 24 March 1977.

66. The seriousness of the discussions was evident in the personnel of the negotiating teams selected by each side. Dr. Ottensmeyer, Chairman of the Board Robert O. Anderson, and J. T. Michelson, an aggressive young Board of Trustees member, spoke for the Lovelace side, and Chief Executive Officer Ray Woodham, the Rev. James Hall (Chairman of the Board, Presbyterian Hospital Center), and Jack Rust, member of the Board, PHC, represented the Presbyterian side.

67. Memorandum, Dr. David J. Ottensmeyer, to Lovelace-Bataan Medical Center Medical Staff, 4 April 1977, in Lovelace Clinic, Medical Staff, Minutes.

68. Lovelace Medical Foundation, Annual Meeting, 1985, Minutes, p. E-22.

stitution. Given its prestige and its newfound vigor of the early eighties, Lovelace was an attractive prospect to a number of regional and national corporations engaged in the health care business. Through the latter part of 1983 and the first months of 1984, Lovelace authorities talked with nearly two dozen health care companies—profit and non-profit—regarding a possible partnership.[69] The list included many of the largest and most influential concerns of the health care industry, among them Hospital Corporation of America (HCA), American Medical International, Health West, and Lutheran Hospital Systems. The discussions were somewhat unusual, since Lovelace was not interested in a "sell-out" to anybody, but rather in a joint venture arrangement which would preserve the distinctiveness of the institution and guarantee the integrity of its research and education programs, while securing access to the financial strength and support essential to survival in the increasingly competitive business of health care. In a report to the Lovelace Foundation's Board of Trustees in March, 1984, Dr. Ottensmeyer spelled out the basic objectives that oriented Lovelace's bargaining with outside interests:

> (1) Lovelace Medical Foundation (LMF) must have sufficient resources and annual revenue to carry on activities central to its mission and goals;
> (2) LMF should manage any resulting healthcare system dependent upon medical staff for operations;
> (3) LMF must have modern ambulatory and acute care facilities and should have equity ownership of that facility;
> (4) Medical education and research must be integrated with healthcare delivery in any resulting organization;
> (5) LMF should have a 50 percent representation in any resulting Board of Directors which appoints the management for the healthcare delivery activities; and
> (6) The jobs and security of the medical staff and employees of LMF must by assured in any organizational rearrangements.[70]

69. Ottensmeyer, interview, 23 August 1985.

70. Lovelace Medical Foundation, Board of Trustees, Annual Meeting, 1985, pp. E-20 and E-21.

The complex and demanding negotiation process bore fruit in June, 1984, when the Lovelace Board of Trustees in special session approved a memorandum of understanding with Hospital Corporation of America. In a novel, pioneering arrangement, the two institutions agreed to create a new entity called the Lovelace Medical Center, Inc. in which HCA would have an 80 percent equity position and the Lovelace Medical Foundation 20 percent. However, the foundation would name 50 percent of the new entity's Board of Directors and have right of approval over the chief executive officer of the new operation. Through the agreement HCA would secure entry into the Albuquerque medical market and would buy into the highly successful Lovelace HMO, a sphere of the health care industry where its experience and expertise were limited. Immediately HCA pledged to begin construction of the critically needed new 243-bed hospital for the Lovelace campus at a projected cost of 43 million dollars plus 6 million dollars for new equipment.[71] For its part Lovelace would get the new hospital it so badly needed and the liquidation of its existing debt, plus a number of other services and advantages available through its giant partner. For instance, through its linkage with HCA Lovelace could expect the economic savings afforded through integration within the group purchasing of its partner. In addition, it could secure capital on better terms than those likely to be available to it as a "stand-alone" institution. And, the partnership with HCA gave the Albuquerque institution access to the managerial and other support systems already developed by the national concern.

On the Lovelace campus there was much anxiety and uncertainty associated with this innovative agreement with the national corporate giant, for it represented a venture into uncharted waters for the Albuquerque medical center, but there was much optimism as well. That confidence in the future was fortified as, beginning with groundbreaking in October, 1985, the new hospital began to take form during the following months. A period of "feeling out" and working out the details of the

71. These were the projected figures in use as of November, 1984.

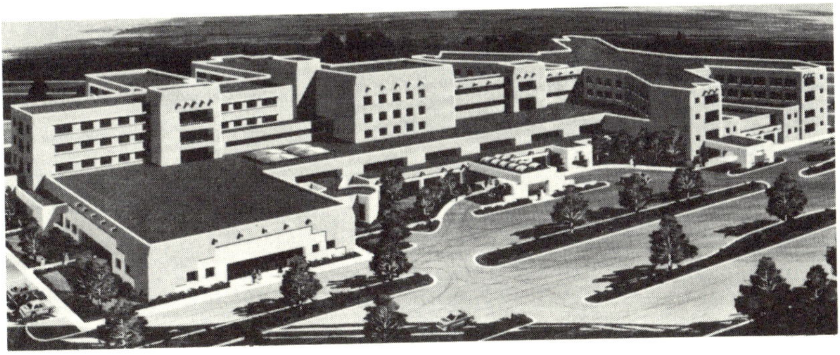

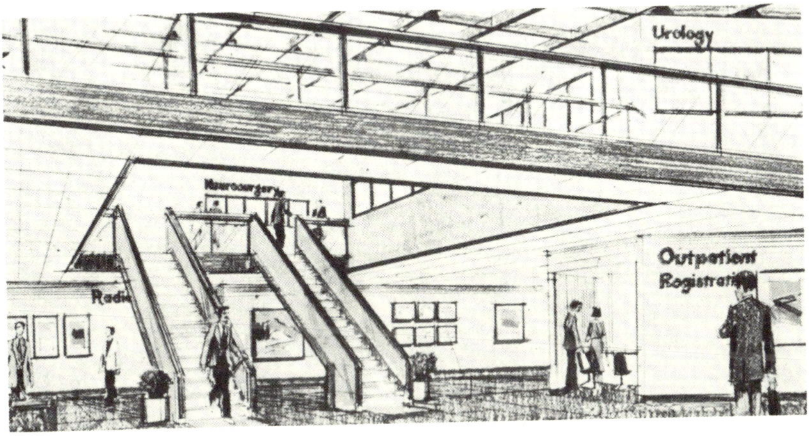

An architectural rendering of the exterior of the Lovelace Medical Center as it will look after completion of the new hospital and education building. Below, an architectural rendering of the new facility's interior.

new joint venture followed the 1 February 1985 effective date of the HCA-Lovelace agreement, but the early working relationship within the new combination was a good and constructive one. The period of adjustment was extended in October, 1986, when additional corporate changes took place. At that time, Lovelace became associated with a second giant of the corporate health-care world, the Equitable Life Assurance Society of the United States. Through the spring and summer of 1986, discussions took place between the Hospital Corporation of America and The Equitable aiming toward creation of a new company called Equicor, a joint venture enterprise intended to offer managed health care and other employee benefit programs on a broad, national scale. HCA's Health Plans Division, of which the Lovelace Health Plan was a part, and the Equitable Group and Health Insurance Company Division of the insurance giant were spun off to form the new company, and the Albuquerque medical complex was aligned within the new entity. These changes at the corporate level were accompanied by managerial changes on Gibson Boulevard, when Dr. Ottensmeyer left Albuquerque to become a senior vice-president of Nashville-based HCA—he remained as chairman of the board of Lovelace Medical Center Inc.—and was succeeded as president and chief executive officer by Dr. Derick Pasternak, an experienced fourteen-year veteran of the Lovelace operation. These transitions, both corporate and managerial, took place without ruffling the work of the thriving Lovelace medical complex, a tribute to the strength and solidity of its structure.

As 1987 neared, the Lovelace institution prepared to celebrate several significant milestones of its history. That year was simultaneously the 65th anniversary of the birth of the Lovelace Clinic, the 40th anniversary of the establishment of the Lovelace Foundation, and the 35th anniversary of the opening of Bataan Hospital. (1987 was also, of course, the year of the opening of the new Lovelace hospital.) It was a natural occasion to consider the accomplishments of the past decades and to contemplate the possibilities of the future. Just as, early in the century, the senior Dr. Lovelace had been forced to relocate and to pioneer in the turbulent milieu of frontier New Mexico, so, too, the institution he founded and nurtured prepared itself for continued service in the shifting circumstances of the end of that same century. Its tradition of pioneering steeled its resolution to challenge the tasks ahead.

Bibliography

I. PRIMARY MATERIALS

This study of Lovelace history rests basically on two sources: the surprisingly complete records of the Lovelace Medical Center itself and the recollections of the people associated with it. (See section III, below, for a list of the people formally interviewed as part of the preparation for this work.) Since the formation of the Lovelace Foundation in 1947, the records of the institution have been carefully preserved, so that the documentary legacy of the Lovelace medical center is physically large and comprehensive in scope. Over the nearly three years spent in researching this book, those records have been identified, collected, and consolidated in one place for the first time. They are presently held in a library-archives room in the Lovelace Medical Foundation building and will eventually be placed in a specially constructed archives room in the new Education Building yet to be built on the Lovelace campus. A special thanks is extended here to the numerous Lovelace administrators, secretaries, and others who preserved through thick and thin their shares of the Lovelace heritage, even when the pressures were strong to clean "that old stuff" from their files and closets. Because of their faithfulness and sense of history, Lovelace can document its past in a way few comparable institutions can.

The primary record collections used in producing this history are

A. Lovelace Medical Foundation records
Annual Education Report (1958–74)
Annual Research Report (1949/50–86) Title varies.
Board of Trustees. Minutes. 21 volumes. 25 September 1947 through 5 April 1986. (Includes Executive Committee minutes.)

B. Bataan Memorial Methodist Hospital records
Annual Report (1952–75) Title varies.
Board of Directors. Minutes. 5 volumes. 10 January 1951 through 30 July 1969.

C. Lovelace Clinic records
Board of Governors. Minutes. 91 volumes. 3 July 1953 through 16 December 1985. (This collection includes correspondence and reports to and from the Board.)
Medical Staff. Minutes. 22 volumes. 28 January 1954 through 2 December 1985. (This collection includes correspondence and reports.)

These record groups constitute the major sources for Lovelace's history, but the institution's archives contain more than 150 other collections, some of them quite large physically and important to the center's history. For example, there are individual records, including file folders on most of the prominent people—physicians, administrators, trustees, and others—associated with the medical center; a large (numbering in the thousands) photograph collection; personal correspondence files, including scattered correspondence of William Randolph Lovelace I, Floyd Odlum, Sam White, Don Kilgore, and others; land and other legal documents; subject files on special issues of importance within the institution's history—such as the restrictive covenant clause, the satellite clinic operations, the health maintenance organization, the major research projects of the Foundation, and much else; administrative records; the personal files of Dr. Kilgore during the five years of his service as president and chief executive officer of the center; personal memorabilia of both Drs. Lovelace; the records of numerous committees within the institution; newspaper clippings scrapbooks; and much else. These collections are in process of final organization.

Other archival collections of use in preparation of this study include the Medical History Archives at the University of New Mexico Medical Center Library, which holds the records of the New Mexico Medical Society and the Bernalillo County Medical Association (now the Greater Albuquerque Medical Association) and a large collection of oral history interviews with New Mexico physicians and other health professionals, many of which shed interesting light on Lovelace history. The Special Collections Department at the University of New Mexico's Main Library holds a complete copy of the territorial archives of the Territory of New Mexico, a Maxwell Land Grant collection, and a small, scattered group of Lovelace materials, all of which were surveyed for this work. The newspaper clippings collection at the Albuquerque Public Library was useful, as was the photograph collection at the Museum of Albuquerque. The files of St. Joseph Hospital produced some pieces of information, particularly regarding Dr. Lovelace I, and the newspaper morgue of the *Albuquerque Journal* provided some help. Outside Albuquerque, miscellaneous materials were secured from the NASA History Office in Washington, D.C.; the library of the New York Academy of Medicine in New York City; the Board of Medical Examiners' office and files in Santa Fe; the archives of the St. Louis University School of Medicine; the Museum of New Mexico in Santa Fe; and the National Library of Medicine in Bethesda, Maryland.

II. BOOKS AND ARTICLES

American Medical Association, Bureau of Medical Economics. *Group Practice.* Chicago: American Medical Association, 1933.

Benford, Robert Joseph. *Doctors in the Sky: The Story of the Aero Medical Association.* Springfield, Illinois: Charles Thomas, 1955.

Boothby, Walter M. and W. Randolph Lovelace II. "Oxygen in Aviation: The Necessity for the Use of Oxygen and a Practical Apparatus for Its Administration to Both Pilots and Passengers." *The Journal of Aviation Medicine* 39 (1938): 172–99.

Caldwell, Guy A. *Early History of the Ochsner Medical Center: The First Twenty-two Years.* Springfield, Illinois: Charles Thomas, 1965.

Carrington, Paul M. "The Climate of New Mexico, Nature's Sanatorium for Consumptives." *New York Medical Journal* 86 (1907): 1–10.

Center for Research in Ambulatory Health Care Administration. *The Organization and Development of a Medical Group Practice.* Cambridge, Mass.: Ballinger Publishing Co., 1976.

Council on Medical Service, American Medical Association. "Survey of Group Practice." *Journal of the American Medical Association* 164 (1957): 1338–48.

Davis, Ellis Arthur, ed. *The Historical Encyclopedia of New Mexico.* 2 volumes. Albuquerque, N.M.: New Mexico Historical Association, 1945.

Dorn, Ronald V., Jr. "The Lovelace Clinic." *Group Practice* 14 (1965): 327–38.

Elliott, Richard G. " 'On a Comet, Always.' A Biography of Dr. W. Randolph Lovelace II." *New Mexico Quarterly* 36 (1966–67): 351–88.

Engle, Eloise and Arnold S. Lott. *Man in Flight: Biomedical Achievements in Aerospace.* Annapolis, Maryland: Leeward Publications, Inc., 1979.

Falkson, Joseph. *HMOs and the Politics of Health System Reform.* Chicago: American Hospital Association, 1980.

Haber, Heinz and Slade Hulbert. *Proceedings of a Symposium on Escape from High Performance Aircraft.* Los Angeles: The Institute of Transportation and Traffic Engineering, UCLA, 1956.

Link, Mae Mills. *Space Medicine in Project Mercury.* Washington: National Aeronautics and Space Administration, 1965.

Loeppky, J. A. and M. L. Riedesel, eds. *Oxygen Transport to Human Tissues: A Symposium in Honor of Dr. U. C. Luft.* New York and Amsterdam: Elsevier Biomedical, 1983.

Long, Esmond R. "Tuberculosis in Modern Society." *Bulletin of the History of Medicine* 27 (1953): 301–19.

Lovelace, William R., I. "Fibrolipoma of Left Labium Majora." *Journal of the American Medical Association* 80 (1923):375–77.

———. "Implantation of a Biliary Fistula into the Gastrointestinal Tract: Case Report and Two Year Follow-Up." *Southwestern Medicine* 16 (1932): 159–64.

———. "The Surgical Treatment of Tuberculosis." *Southwestern Medicine* 10 (1926): 472–77.

———, Walter A. Gekler, H. P. Rankin, and V. J. Weigel. "Tuberculous Cavitation of the Lung: Mechanical Factors in Its Genesis and Combined Chermotherapeutic and Surgical Treatment." *Journal of the American Medical Association* 82 (1924): 457–63.

Lovelace, W. Randolph, II, and A. H. Schwichtenberg. "Space Medicine and the Future." *Astronautics* 8 (1961): 58–59, 98, 100, 102.

———, A. H. Schwichtenberg, Ulrich Luft, and Robert R. Secrest. "Selection and Maintenance Program for Astronauts for the National Aeronautics and Space Administration." *Aerospace Medicine* 33 (1962): 667–84.

Martin, Edward T. "The Hero of High-Altitude Flight." *Air Line Pilot* 52 (1983): 22–24, 38–39.

Mayo, Charles W. *Mayo: The Story of My Family and My Career.* Garden City, New York: Doubleday and Co., 1968.

McAlavy, Don. "Fort Sumner Country" in *Curry County, New Mexico.* Dallas: High Plains Historical Foundation, 1978.

McClellan, Roger O. "Twenty-five Years of Lovelace Research in Inhalation Toxicology." *New Mexico Journal of Science* 26 (1986): 330–45.

McFarland, Ross A. *Human Factors in Air Transportation: Occupational Health and Safety.* New York: McGraw-Hill, 1953.

Newell, Homer E. *Beyond the Atmosphere: Early Years of Space Science.* The NASA History Series. Washington: Scientific and Technical Information Branch, National Aeronautics and Space Administration, 1980.

Pomrinse, S. David. "The Growth and Development of Medical Group Practice." *Journal of the American Medical Association* 177 (1961): 765–70.

Rogers, Frank B. "The Rise and Decline of the Altitude Therapy of Tuberculosis." *Bulletin of the History of Medicine* 43 (1969): 1–16.

Rorem, C. Rufus. *Private Group Clinics.* Chicago: University of Chicago Press, 1931.

Roth, Emmanuel M., ed. *Compendium of Human Responses to the Aerospace Environment.* 4 volumes. Albuquerque, N.M.: Lovelace Foundation for Medical Education and Research, 1968.

Schwichtenberg, A. H., Donald D. Flickinger, and W. Randolph Lovelace II. "Development and Use of Medical Machine Record Cards in Astronaut Selection." *U.S. Armed Forces Medical Journal* 10 (1959): 1324–51.

Soule, Samuel D. *Medicine in St. Louis Medical Schools in the Nineteenth Century.* St. Louis: William Washington Graves Lecture Series, 1978.

Spidle, Jake W. "Albuquerque's Lovelace Clinic: A Tradition of Excellence." *New Mexico Journal of Science* 26 (1986): 322–29.

———. "A Place to Serve: Albuquerque's Lovelace Clinic, 1922 to the Present." *Postgraduate Medicine* 78 (1985): 16–24.

———. *Doctors of Medicine in New Mexico: A History of Health and Medical Practice, 1886–1986.* Albuquerque, N.M.: University of New Mexico Press, 1986.

Starr, Paul. *The Social Transformation of American Medicine.* New York: Basic Books, 1982.

"Sutures and Sixguns." *Forum Magazine* [Lovelace-Bataan Medical Center] 1 (1974): 1–4.

Terris, Milton. "Origins and Growth of Group Practice." *Bulletin of the New York Academy of Medicine* 44 (1968): 1277–81.

Thomas, Shirley. *Men of Space: Profiles of the Leaders in Space Research, Development, and Exploration.* Philadelphia and New York: Chilton Co., 1965.

Warden, Carol A. *A Tradition of Medical Progress: History of the Santa Barbara Medical Foundation Clinic.* Santa Barbara, California: Santa Barbara Medical Foundation Clinic, 1985.

Wasserman, Fred W. and Michael C. Miller. *Building a Group Practice.* Springfield, Illinois: Charles C. Thomas, 1973.

White, Clayton S. "The Lovelace Years" in J. A. Loeppky and M. L.

Riedesel, eds., *Oxygen Transport to Human Tissues: A Symposium in Honor of Dr. U. C. Luft* (New York and Amsterdam: Elsevier Biomedical, 1983), 3–12.

——— and Otis O. Benson, eds. *Physics and Medicine of the Upper Atmosphere: A Study of the Aeropause.* Albuquerque, N.M.: University of New Mexico Press, 1952.

Wilds, John. *Ochsner's: An Informal History of the South's Largest Private Medical Center.* Baton Rouge: Louisiana State University Press, 1985.

"William R. Lovelace, M.D." *The Lovelace Clinic Review* 1 (1962): 96–102.

Wolfe, Tom. *The Right Stuff.* New York: Farrar, Straus, Giroux, 1979.

III. INTERVIEWS

(All interviews were with the author, except as noted.)

Adler, Stuart W., M.D. Albuquerque, New Mexico, 21 September 1982.

Anderson, Robert O. Albuquerque, New Mexico, 30 August 1985.

Badger, Demarious, M.D. Albuquerque, New Mexico, 2 September 1983.

Barol, Samuel R., M.D. Albuquerque, New Mexico, 24 March 1986.

Bivens, Melvin, M.D. Albuquerque, New Mexico, 1 May 1986.

Campbell, Jack. Albuquerque, New Mexico, 25 October 1985.

Chiffelle, Thomas L., M.D. Albuquerque, New Mexico, 23 March 1985.

Cornish, P. G., III, M.D. Albuquerque, New Mexico, 21 November 1983.

Cramer, Oliver S., M.D. Albuquerque, New Mexico, 3 October 1984.

Derbyshire, Robert C., M.D. Interview with Dr. Peter Olch and the author. Albuquerque, New Mexico, 9 October 1982.

Dornacker, John. Albuquerque, New Mexico, 7 March 1985.

Eurich, Alvin. Interview with Merle Tucker and the author. New York City, New York, 5 January 1985.

Fischer, Arthur, M.D. Albuquerque, New Mexico, 21 January 1985.

Fishback, Charles F., M.D. Albuquerque, New Mexico, 4 June 1985.

Fulcher, Joe R. G. Albuquerque, New Mexico, 11 December 1986.

Gwinn, A. Clay, M.D. Carlsbad, New Mexico, 11 March 1985.

Hardy, William R., M.D. Albuquerque, New Mexico, 23 August 1984.

Johnson, Earl D. Interview with Merle Tucker and the author. Greenwich, Connecticut, 6 January 1985.

Kilgore, Donald E., M.D. Albuquerque, New Mexico, 18 November 1985.

Lassetter, Edgar L., M.D. Albuquerque, New Mexico, 8 August 1985.
Levin, Louis, M.D. Albuquerque, New Mexico, 19 September 1984.
Luft, Ulrich C., M.D. Albuquerque, New Mexico, 11 October 1985.
MacQuigg, Rodger, M.D. Albuquerque, New Mexico, 10 October 1984.
Marshall, I. J., M.D. Roswell, New Mexico, 15 August 1983.
Marshall, Ralph. Interview with Dr. Peter Olch and the author. Albuquerque, New Mexico, 7 October 1982.
Massey, Robert U., M.D. Interview with Merle Tucker and the author. Farmington, Connecticut, 4 January 1985.
McCarthy, Jack, M.D. Albuquerque, New Mexico, 7 March 1986.
McClellan, Roger O., D.V.M. Albuquerque, New Mexico, 1 August 1985.
McKay, Horace. Albuquerque, New Mexico, 9 December 1985.
McKinnon, D. Angus, M.D. Albuquerque, New Mexico, 25 October 1984.
Michelson, J. T. Albuquerque, New Mexico, 15 September 1985.
Ottensmeyer, David J., M.D. Albuquerque, New Mexico, 23 August 1985.
Pasternak, Derick, M.D. Albuquerque, New Mexico, 21 April 1986.
Savage, George. Albuquerque, New Mexico, 8 February 1985.
Schmitt, Harrison "Jack." Albuquerque, New Mexico, 8 May 1986.
Schwichtenberg, A. H., M.D. Albuquerque, New Mexico, 20 February 1985.
Simms, Albert G., III, M.D. Albuquerque, New Mexico, 17 May 1984.
Slayton, Donald K. "Deke". Houston, Texas, 12 May 1986.
Smith, C. R. Interview with Merle Tucker and the author. Washington, D.C., 7 January 1985.
Turner, Robert S., M.D. Albuquerque, New Mexico, 31 March 1986.
Twiest, Melvin, M.D. Albuquerque, New Mexico, 22 September 1986.
White, Clayton S., M.D. Albuquerque, New Mexico, 14 October 1985.
Womack, Carroll L., M.D. Carlsbad, New Mexico, 12 March 1985.

IV. UNPUBLISHED MATERIAL

Columbia University. Oral History Research Office. "The Reminiscences of Dr. William Randolph Lovelace II." 1960. Transcript.
Johnson, Judie. "The Lovelace Medical Center." Unpublished paper, University of New Mexico History Department, November, 1981.
Lovelace, William Randolph, II. "Oxygen in Aviation and Surgery: A New and Practical Apparatus for Its Administration." M.S. thesis, University of Minnesota, 1939.
McClellan, Roger O. "The Inhalation Toxicology Research Institute." Unpublished manuscript, 16 January 1981.

Index